OXFORD MEDICAL PUBLICATIONS

Sex therapy: a practical guide

SEX THERAPY:

A practical guide

KEITH HAWTON

Consultant Psychiatrist, Warneford Hospital, Oxford;
Clinical Lecturer in Psychiatry
University of Oxford

OXFORD
OXFORD UNIVERSITY PRESS 1985
NEW YORK TORONTO

Oxford University Press, Walton Street, Oxford OX2 6DP
London New York Toronto
Delhi Bombay Calcutta Madras Karachi
Kuala Lumpur Singapore Hong Kong Tokyo
Nairobi Dar es Salaam Cape Town
Melbourne Auckland
and associated companies in
Beirut Berlin Ibadan Mexico City Nicosia

Oxford is a trade mark of Oxford University Press

Published in the United States
by Oxford University Press, New York

British Library Cataloguing in Publication Data
Hawton, Keith
    Sex therapy: a practical guide.—(Oxford
    medical publications)
    1. Sex therapy
    I. Title
    616.6'906   RC556
ISBN 0-19-261413-4

Typeset by DMB Typesetting, Oxford
Printed in Great Britain by
The Thetford Press, Thetford, Norfolk

Acknowledgements

I am deeply indebted to John Bancroft for first introducing me to this field, and to Lorna and Phil Sarrell who, some years ago, shared with me the benefits of their extensive experience of sex therapy in the USA. Many of the ideas expressed in this book have developed out of discussions with these and other colleagues, especially the numerous trainees from psychiatry, clinical psychology, marriage guidance, and social work who have attended my supervision groups during the past nine years. I am extremely grateful for the critical comments on an early draft of this book that were provided by José Catalán, Melanie Fennell, Diane James, Susan Harrison, Elena Snow, and Christopher Watson. The typing of the various drafts of the manuscript was carried out willingly and conscientiously by Triona Baillie, Diana Broun, Pat English, and Beverley Haggis. Lastly, and most importantly, I thank my wife, Joan, who sustained my motivation, and made numerous suggestions about both the content and style of the text, despite the demands of a young family and her own professional commitments.

Oxford, 1984   Keith Hawton

Contents

1

Introduction

The history of therapeutic approaches to helping people with
sexual problems provides a fascinating story. It has reflected
overall trends in therapeutic methods introduced for the treatment of a wide variety of psychological problems. Thus the
emphasis has shifted from the extremes of either psychoanalytical
or physical treatments to briefer and more directive therapy based
on modern psychological principles and our improved understanding of sexuality. In addition, the innovations in this field
have paralleled the enormous changes in public attitudes to sexuality which were especially marked during the 1960s and early
1970s.

Although there is ample room and much need for further improving the range and effectiveness of treatment methods, sexual
medicine and especially sex therapy are established as major fields
of therapeutic endeavour. Nowadays, effective help can be offered
to most people who seek help for sexual problems. This relatively
favourable situation has evolved during little more than the past
decade. It has been based on a rather disjointed series of historical
developments, as has been the case with many other psychological
therapies.

Until quite recently, sexual dysfunctions were regarded as
symptoms of deep-seated disturbances of personality originating
from early childhood experiences. Freud (1949) postulated that
disturbances in maturation through the various phases of childhood sexuality which interfered with the normal development of
child-parent relationships were the root of sexual problems. On
the basis of this theory, sexual dysfunctions were regarded as

relatively resistant to therapy. If available, treatment usually consisted of lengthy psychoanalysis or insight-orientated psychotherapy, which was always provided on an individual basis. Because of the vast amount of therapeutic time and considerable expense involved, such treatment was only available for a small minority of people. Also, as far as can be gathered from the literature, the results of treatment were poor and a very pessimistic attitude towards sexual dysfunction prevailed (Bergler 1951).

A change in this attitude began to occur following two important developments during the late 1950s and early 1960s. The first was the introduction of behaviour therapy. In 1958, Wolpe suggested the method of systematic desensitization as a therapeutic approach to erectile dysfunction and other sexual difficulties. Several reports subsequently appeared, usually based on the treatment of only a few patients, in which behaviour therapy methods had been used relatively successfully to overcome sexual problems, including 'frigidity' (Lazarus 1963; Brady 1966), vaginismus (Haslam 1965), and erectile dysfunction (Friedman 1968). In addition, there was an isolated report of a novel approach, now called the 'stop-start technique', for the treatment of premature ejaculation (Semans 1956). The introduction of these more directive approaches represented a vast conceptual shift from the psychoanalytical stance mentioned earlier, because the focus of treatment was now current behaviour and its maintenance rather than distant and hypothetical causes for sexual problems.

The second development, which occurred on a much smaller scale, but was nevertheless important, was the introduction in the UK of a brief psychotherapeutic approach, based on the teaching of Michael Balint (Balint 1957; Balint and Balint 1961), for the management of the sexual problems of women. This development, which is described in a fascinating book by Friedman (1962), is of particular interest because it incorporated both brief psychotherapeutic strategies and more behaviourally orientated techniques in a way that has become the hallmark of modern sex therapy. For example, in the treatment of vaginismus, a vaginal examination by a woman doctor was used for therapeutic purposes in order to encourage the patient to talk about her anxieties and fears concerning vaginal penetration by her partner.

These were then explored more fully in order to try and help the woman understand and overcome them. One important respect in which both this approach and the early behavioural methods differed from modern sex therapy was that treatment was focused on the individual rather than the couple, with partners excluded from the treatment session.

The most important development in this field, which represented a watershed between the earlier therapies and what is now available for people with sexual problems, was the publication in 1970 of the book *Human sexual inadequacy* by Masters and Johnson. This described a very different approach, based partly on extensive studies of sexual response in men and women (Masters and Johnson 1966). What Masters and Johnson developed, although they themselves do not describe it quite in these terms, was a unique combination of behavioural, psychotherapeutic, and educational elements that provided a relatively straightforward approach to the management of the sexual problems of couples. The focus of therapy became the couple and the relationship between the partners.

The results of treatment reported by Masters and Johnson for a very large series of couples were quite remarkable and, although they have since been subject to much criticism, were responsible for the enormous enthusiasm that rapidly developed in the United States and elsewhere for 'sex therapy', as it has since become known. As with many other psychological treatments, the initial enthusiasm of its advocates was based on virtually no research evidence, except for the results reported by Masters and Johnson. This enthusiasm unfortunately attracted some people who had little or no previous therapeutic experience and who saw sex therapy as providing an opportunity for financial exploitation of patients. This unwelcome development, which was far more prevalent in the USA than elsewhere, resulted in some discrediting of sex therapy. In addition, because the Masters and Johnson approach was designed for couples, individuals with sexual problems were relatively neglected. As will become apparent later in this book, this situation has recently changed such that effective therapeutic approaches are now available both for couples and for individuals.

The initial enthusiasm for sex therapy has been tempered, and a more realistic attitude currently prevails. The value and limits of sex therapy are now more firmly based on empirical findings. However, as will become apparent in subsequent chapters, there still remain considerable research needs in this field.

Several books on sex therapy have now been published. The original impetus for writing this book, however, was that there did not appear to be a practical guide for therapists giving a straight-forward account of the therapeutic approaches now available for helping people with sexual problems. This book is intended to provide both detailed guidance for those wishing to begin sex therapy, and an up-to-date account for those simply wishing to become more familiar with the field. It is hoped that experienced therapists will also find the book of interest.

An important advantage of the current therapeutic approaches to sexual problems is that, by and large, they do not require an exhaustive training in a particular specialist field. Sexual prob-lems can be managed by people from a variety of disciplines, including, for example, psychiatrists, clinical psychologists, general practitioners, social workers, nurses, obstetricians and gynaecologists, and family planning doctors. In addition, many marriage guidance counsellors are now able to offer sex therapy as well as general marital counselling. It is to people in all these, and other disciplines, that this book is directed, hence the general term 'therapist' which is used throughout. While the book is intended to be a detailed practical therapeutic guide, it is recom-mended that novices to the field should try to use it in conjunc-tion with supervision from an experienced therapist.

Before starting therapy it is essential to gain a sound under-standing of sexual anatomy and sexual response. This is therefore the focus of the next chapter. Following that, Part I is devoted to consideration of the nature of sexual problems (Chapter 3), their prevalence and effects (Chapter 4), and their causes (Chapter 5). The description of the causes of sexual problems in Chapter 5 should convey the extensive range of aetiological factors, and, in particular, their interactions.

The rest of the book (Part II) is concerned with therapy. The description of therapeutic approaches for helping couples with sexual problems is divided into the stages of assessment (Chap-ter 6), explaining the problem to the couple (Chapter 7), the behavioural components of therapy or 'homework assignments' (Chapter 8), psychotherapeutic aspects of therapy (Chapter 9), educational measures (Chapter 10), helping with general relationship issues (Chapter 11), and the termination of treatment (Chapter 12). An important reason for writing this book was the paucity of straightforward descriptions in the literature of what a therapist can do when couples encounter difficulties in trying to carry out their homework assignments. The description of psychotherapeutic procedures in Chapter 9 provides a simple approach that can be used by therapists who do not necessarily have extensive prior experience of psychotherapy. Similarly, the educational measures described in Chapter 10 are quite easy to apply, provided the therapist has a reasonable understanding of sexual anatomy and response.

The final chapter concerning sex therapy with couples (Chapter 13) is a brief review of the main research findings currently available to substantiate the approach to sex therapy which has been described in the earlier chapters.

Chapter 14 describes the ways in which sex therapy has been developed in order to meet the needs of other patients, including those without partners, those whose problems do not necessitate a full programme of sex therapy, and those who have sexual problems associated with physical disorders. The provision of therapy in groups is also outlined.

Finally, Chapter 15 includes a general appraisal of the current state of the field, and some of the main areas for future clinical and research developments.

This book has been written in a spirit of therapeutic optimism, trying to convey to the reader the great variety of ways in which sexuality may be impaired and the innovative approaches which now enable us to offer help to people with sexual problems. Wherever possible, reference has been made to substantiating research findings; where such evidence has not been available, reliance on the clinical experience of the author and many other people has been necessary.

2

Sexual anatomy
and sexual response

INTRODUCTION

Anyone who wishes to help people with sexual problems must have adequate knowledge and understanding of sexual anatomy, physiology, and response. This is the subject of this chapter. Detailed description of human sexual anatomy has long been available in standard general textbooks of anatomy. In 1933 Dickinson published his book *Human sex anatomy*, which was updated in 1949 in his *Atlas of human sex anatomy*. Even today the latter serves as a very valuable reference book. Additional information concerning sexual anatomy, especially the changes which occur during sexual arousal, has been provided by Masters and Johnson (1966).

The situation with regard to sexual physiology is rather different. In spite of a considerable research effort in this field, we still remain relatively ignorant concerning, for example, the precise roles that sex hormones play in human sexuality and, of more concern to us here, what roles they might have in the development of sexual dysfunction, especially in women.

We owe a large debt to Masters and Johnson for their work on the sexual responses of men and women (Masters and Johnson 1966). Their studies have contributed much to our current understanding of the changes which occur during sexual arousal. However, many people are unaware that Kinsey and his colleagues, apart from their studies of the epidemiology of sexuality (p. 45), also carried out observational and photographic studies of sexual arousal in men and women. This aspect of their research was kept secret until publication of their volume on female sexuality (Kinsey *et al.* 1953) for fear of official and public disapproval. Masters and Johnson (1966) have acknowledged the efforts of Kinsey and colleagues in this area, which provided a basis for their own, more sophisticated laboratory studies of sexual response. However, their own work has not been without controversy. In Belliveau and Richter's (1970) summary of the first two major books by Masters and Johnson we learn of the unfavourable and even hostile attitudes shown to their work by colleagues and academic journals. Fortunately, their pioneering efforts continued and eventually provided a basis for the development of the therapeutic procedures which have revolutionized the management of sexual problems.

Masters and Johnson (1966) described a four-stage model of sexual response. As they themselves emphasized, the four stages represent an arbitrary subdivision of the changes that occur during sexual response. However, their model has largely retained its popularity and will therefore be used here. In summary, the first stage of sexual response is the *excitement phase*, in which sexual arousal develops in response to sexual stimulation, which may be of any kind, including fantasy as well as physical stimulation. If sexual arousal intensifies, the second stage, or *plateau phase*, is reached from which the individual can experience orgasm. The third stage is the *orgasmic phase*, in which there is involuntary release of sexual tension, usually associated with pleasure, and also in men by ejaculation. After orgasm, or either of the first two stages if orgasm does not occur, sexual tension is dissipated in the fourth stage, or *resolution phase*, in which the bodily changes that have accompanied sexual arousal return to normal.

Kaplan (1974) put forward a somewhat different, biphasic model. She suggested that sexual response consists of two relatively independent components, namely: (i) genital vasocongestion producing male erection and female vaginal congestion and lubrication, followed by (ii) reflex muscular contractions which constitute orgasm. The primary basis for her biphasic model was that the first component is largely under the influence of the parasympathetic nervous system and the second is largely mediated via the sympathetic nervous system. She also suggested that the two components are differentially affected by drugs, trauma, and age. Kaplan's model has not proved as useful as that of Masters and Johnson in conceptualizing sexual response. However, in further publications in 1977 and 1979, Kaplan added a third component to her biphasic model, namely that of 'sexual desire'. While not being essential to our understanding here of normal sexual response, this is an important concept when one attempts to classify and describe the different forms of sexual dysfunction (Chapter 3).

In the rest of this chapter the sexual anatomy, physiology, and response of men and women will be considered separately. However, it is worth emphasizing that some of the most surprising results of studies of sexual response have been the similarities that have been found between the two sexes. This description will only be a brief summary, restricted to the needs of the practising sex therapist. Those readers who wish for more detailed information, especially with regard to sexual physiology and response, are referred to the original work by Masters and Johnson (1966) and to recent reviews by Bancroft (1980) and Levin (1980).

FEMALE SEXUAL ANATOMY

Although this section will largely be concerned with the genitals, we must not forget that the whole of the body is important in sexual behaviour. Apart from the obvious importance of breasts in sexual attraction and stimulation, many other parts of the body may be the source of sexual pleasure. The non-genital aspects of sexuality are the focus of the early stages of sex therapy (p. 128).

External genitals

A woman's external genitals consist of the labia majora, the clitoris, the labia minora, the urethral opening, and the entrance to vagina (Fig. 2.1). The appearance of the genitals can vary considerably from one woman to another; this can sometimes be a source of worry which may be uncovered during sex therapy (p. 218). When a woman is not sexually aroused the labia majora usually meet, providing protection for the labia minora, vagina and urethral opening.

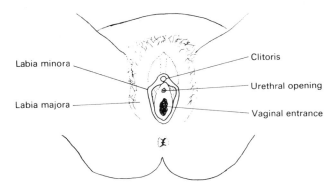

Fig. 2.1 Female external genitals

The clitoris is a very similar structure to the penis, except that it is much smaller and does not contain the urethra. It lies mostly under the clitoral hood. The clitoris consists of a shaft and a head or glans. The whole structure, but especially the head, is highly sensitive. During sexual stimulation the clitoris becomes engorged.

The labia minora (or vaginal lips) lie on either side of the vaginal entrance and join just below the clitoris. They are richly supplied with blood vessels, and become engorged and change in colour during sexual arousal. The urethral opening, which is connected by a short urethra to the bladder, lies between the clitoris and the vaginal entrance.

Internal genitals

These consist of the vagina, cervix, uterus, Fallopian tubes, and ovaries (Fig. 2.2). Again there are considerable differences between one woman and another, especially in relation to age and whether a woman has given birth. As can be seen in Fig. 2.2, the vagina in the non-aroused woman is a potential space, rather than a tube. It is approximately 10 cm (4 in) long. The first third of the vagina from its entrance is very sensitive, whereas most of the rest of the vagina is only supplied by pressure nerve receptors and therefore is largely insensitive. Recent research, however, has suggested that part of the anterior wall of the vagina may be highly sensitive (see below). The vagina is capable of considerable expansion. The lining of the vagina is a mucosal surface (like the inside of

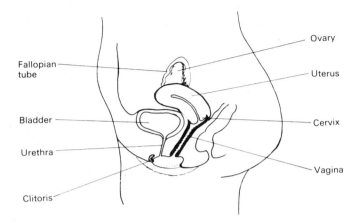

Fig. 2.2 Female internal genitals

the mouth), and the whole of the vagina is richly supplied with blood vessels. An early sign of sexual arousal is the appearance of fluid on the surface of the vagina. This acts as a lubricant to allow smooth and painless entry and movement of the penis during sexual intercourse.

Mention should be made of the Grafenberg or 'G' spot, and female ejaculation, both of which have recently attracted considerable interest (Ladas *et al.* 1982). The Grafenberg spot is a small sensitive area in the anterior wall of the vagina, stimulation of which is said to be responsible for orgasms which occur without any form of clitoral stimulation, as may be the case during sexual intercourse. Evidence has been found for the existence of a specially sensitive area in the vagina of some women (Goldberg *et al.* 1983), although whether stimulation of this area may trigger orgasm is unclear. A more controversial suggestion is that orgasm induced by stimulation of the Grafenberg spot is associated with 'ejaculation' from the urethra of small amounts of fluid (Ladas *et al.* 1982), possibly produced by vestigial glands homologous to the prostate gland in men. Some women do appear to pass a small amount of fluid from the urethra at orgasm (Goldberg *et al.* 1983). However, it is uncertain whether or not this fluid is simply urine. The possible association of such fluid emission with stimulation of the Grafenberg spot also remains unproven.

The cervix is the part of the uterus which protrudes into the vagina. It has an opening, or cervical os. The uterus is a pear-shaped muscular organ which is usually tipped forwards in the pelvis (anteverted). However, in a substantial minority of women it is tipped backwards (retroverted). The two Fallopian tubes enter at the corners of the uterus. Their other openings are near the ovaries.

In addition to the genital structures mentioned so far, there are also pelvic muscles which have special relevance to sexuality. These are the muscles of the pelvic floor. There are three main groups of muscles, all of which are involved in the muscular contractions during orgasm (see Table 2.1). However, they are also important in other ways. Spasm of the muscles surrounding the vaginal entrance is responsible for the condition called 'vaginismus' (p. 33). Training a woman to develop control over these muscles, using the Kegel exercises (p. 218), is one component in the management of both vaginismus and orgasmic dysfunction. We need not dwell on the names of all the muscle groups; sex therapists usually refer only to the 'pubo-coccygeus muscles' which surround the vagina. Although in strict anatomical terms these also include another group of muscles, it will be sufficient for our purposes to refer subsequently only to this muscle group.

FEMALE SEXUAL PHYSIOLOGY AND RESPONSE

The four-stage model of Masters and Johnson (1966) will be used in describing sexual response. However, in taking a wider view of normal sexuality and, later, of sexual problems, it is most important also to include *sexual interest, libido,* or *desire*; these terms are often used interchangeably. Sexual interest, which is the term which will mostly be used here, is a person's general level of interest in sexuality. Although difficult to quantify, sexual interest is reflected in willingness to seek opportunities for sexual contact, the occurrence of sexual thoughts or fantasies, and the frequency of sexual activity, including masturbation as well as that involving a partner. A woman's level of sexual interest may be affected by many factors, especially the nature of her current relationship, her age, her attitudes towards sexuality, and her hormonal status, including, at least in some women, the stage of her menstrual cycle. Many factors may have adverse effects on sexual interest (Chapter 5).

The stages of female sexual response are shown schematically in Fig. 2.3, which is based on Masters and Johnson (1966). A large variety of responses have been observed. Those which are shown (A, B, and C) represent three common patterns. The first (A) represents the response cycle of a woman who passes through all four stages, including orgasm. The second (B) is that of a woman who becomes highly aroused but does not reach orgasm. The third (C) is typical of the rapid response cycle which might occur during masturbation.

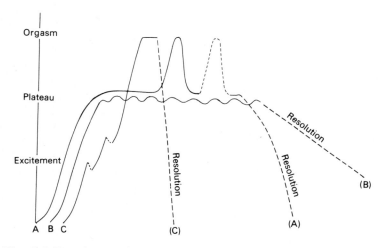

Fig. 2.3 Female sexual response

Some of the physiological and anatomical changes in various parts of the body during the four stages of sexual response are summarized in Table 2.1 at the end of this chapter. We will now focus our attention largely on changes in the genitals during sexual arousal, mindful of factors which are of particular relevance to sex therapy.

Excitement phase

This refers to the anatomical and physiological responses to sexually stimulating activity or thoughts, from the point of earliest arousal to that of high sexual excitement. Most of the changes which occur result from an increase in the flow of blood to the genital organs, and local changes in the blood vessels in these organs. These cause vaginal engorgement and lubrication. There are several important facts about this phase which are relevant to clinical practice.

First, the source of vaginal lubrication (the vaginal mucosal lining) is entirely intravaginal. Because the fluid may remain inside the vagina (unless brought to the vaginal opening with a finger or as a result of heavy lubrication), sometimes one or both partners erroneously assumes that, because the vaginal entrance is dry, the woman is not aroused.

Secondly, as illustrated in response cycle C in Fig. 2.3, although the physiological changes during sexual excitement may proceed steadily if sexual stimulation continues, a woman's *subjective* experience is that of a series of waves of increasing and decreasing sexual arousal or tension. This can be important for the woman who is having difficulty in becoming aroused, because she may become anxious when she feels a wave of arousal fading away. Her anxiety may then inhibit further arousal.

Thirdly, the speed and intensity of changes during the excitement phase will vary greatly between one sexual experience and another in the same woman. During masturbation the excitement phase is often rapid, as is the whole sexual response cycle (C). Some women are able to reach orgasm within two minutes of starting to masturbate. This is in sharp contrast to the widely held belief that women are always much slower to respond than men. Finally, the clitoris is often acutely sensitive during this phase such that many women find direct contact with the clitoral head painful.

Plateau phase

This is the stage of high sexual arousal or tension, during which there is usually some levelling off of arousal. It is also the stage which precedes the threshold level of arousal necessary to trigger orgasm. The duration of this phase varies considerably. One important change that occurs is the retraction of the shaft and glans of the clitoris so that the structure withdraws fully under the clitoral hood and lies up against the pubic symphysis. Sometimes a woman's partner will mistakenly assume that this apparent shrinkage or disappearance of the clitoris means that the woman has ceased to be aroused.

Orgasm

Orgasm appears to be preceded by a sense of 'orgasmic inevitability'. It is probably triggered by a neural reflex arc in response to extreme genital vasocongestion. Orgasm is associated with pleasant sensations which may vary greatly in intensity from one occasion to another. The pubo-coccygeus muscles contract rhythmically during orgasm, the number of contractions varying between 5 and 15. Not all women are aware of these contractions.

One important conclusion that Masters and Johnson (1966) reached was that there is no physiological difference between an orgasm that is the result of indirect clitoral stimulation during sexual intercourse, and one that occurs in response to direct clitoral stimulation. This finding went some way to quashing the claim by psychoanalysts, which had dominated the field of female sexuality for many years, that a 'vaginal orgasm' was superior, in the sense of signifying greater sexual maturity, to a 'clitoral orgasm'.

The sexual response cycle of women does not appear to include a refractory period, which is a characteristic of male sexual response (p. 21). Thus, some women are able to experience a second orgasm soon after the first, without loss of arousal, and, furthermore, may be able in the same way to experience more than two orgasms. However, this by no means applies to all women. Also the number of orgasms a woman experiences may bear no relation to her degree of sexual satisfaction. It is also common for a woman to experience no orgasm in spite of reaching a state of high sexual arousal (B in Fig. 2.3). Some women report that they experience less need to have an orgasm during every session of lovemaking than appears to be true of their partners; whether this is physiologically or culturally determined is unclear. However, very often it is a woman's partner who requires her to experience orgasm in order to satisfy *his* performance anxieties; such psychological pressure can spoil the woman's sexual enjoyment. On the other hand, there are many women who are never or rarely able to achieve orgasm, and for whom this is very distressing (p. 33).

Resolution

During this phase the anatomical and physiological changes that occurred during the three earlier phases are reversed until they return to the normal unaroused state. This is usually accompanied by a sense of relaxation and well-being. It is a phase of great importance in sexual relationships because, while very high sexual arousal and orgasm are often highly personal experiences, this is a time when a couple can share their feelings for each other and experience a unique sense of closeness, assisted by the extreme relaxation that accompanies rapid loss of muscle tone. On the other hand, if the partners quickly shut themselves off from each other, this can result in feelings of rejection which may tarnish the whole sexual experience.

The speed with which resolution occurs varies according to the nature of the rest of the sexual response cycle, and other factors, such as age and whether or not the woman has had children. If, as is often the case during masturbation, the sexual response cycle has been rapid then resolution is also rapid. If the cycle has been more prolonged then resolution occurs more slowly; resolution also takes longer if a state of high sexual tension has been reached but orgasm has not occurred.

Neurological basis of female sexual response
The neurological basis of a woman's sexual response is less well understood than that of men. At present it is assumed that the peripheral nerves necessary for genital engorgement, vaginal lubrication, and orgasm correspond to those which control erection and ejaculation (p. 21).

Hormonal aspects of female sexual behaviour
The main hormones relevant to female sexuality are, first, *oestrogens* and, possibly, *progesterone*, which are produced by the ovaries under the control of *gonadotrophins* (luteinizing hormone (LH) and follicle stimulating hormone (FSH) secreted by the pituitary gland; and, secondly, *androgens*, which are produced by both the adrenal cortex and the ovaries. There are very marked variations in the circulating levels of oestrogens and progesterone during the menstrual cycle, with smaller variations in androgen levels around a mid-cycle or ovulatory peak. Although considerable uncertainty still surrounds the role of these hormones in female sexuality (Sanders and Bancroft 1982), it appears that oestrogens

are necessary to maintain the vaginal mucosa in its normal state, and to allow the full vaginal response, including engorgement and lubrication, to sexual stimulation. Androgens are probably important determinants of sexual interest and of a woman's desire to initiate sexual activity (p. 82). The role, if any, of progesterone in female sexuality is obscure.

The effects of ageing on female sexuality

Some of the general effects of ageing on sexuality are discussed later (p. 66). It has been suggested that women attain peak levels of sexual arousability during their thirties. The main effects of ageing on female sexuality are associated with the changes which occur at the menopause. An important factor is the marked reduction in circulating oestrogen found in the post-menopausal woman. As noted above, oestrogens are important in the maintenance of the normal state of the vagina and in sexual response. The post-menopausal vaginal mucosa undergoes thinning. In addition, there is reduction of lubrication during sexual arousal. These factors can cause discomfort during sexual intercourse. There is some evidence that if a woman remains sexually active these changes are less marked. Ageing also results in some shrinkage of the vagina and of the labia minora. The sensitivity of the vagina is reduced. Shrinkage of the hood of the clitoris results, somewhat paradoxically, in greater exposure of the clitoris to stimulation during foreplay and sexual intercourse.

In addition to reduced vaginal lubrication and clitoral engorgement during sexual arousal, breast swelling and nipple erection (Table 2.1) are also less marked. A woman may experience orgasm less often, the multi-orgasmic woman may have fewer orgasms, the intensity of orgasm may be reduced, and the muscular component of orgasm may be limited because of atrophy of the perineal muscles. Finally, the resolution phase becomes more rapid.

As discussed later (p. 66), a number of general effects of ageing, which will vary widely from individual to individual, are also of importance with regard to sexuality of the older woman. These include obesity, arthritis, and physical illnesses and their treatments. However, having noted what are largely deleterious effects of ageing on a woman's sexuality, it is encouraging to find that many women continue to be sexually active and enjoy sexual intercourse until their sixties, seventies, and even eighties. Thus, for example, Persson (1980) in Sweden found that 16 per cent of 266 women aged 70 remained sexually active. For the 91 women in this study who were married the figure was 36 per cent.

MALE SEXUAL ANATOMY

It is just as necessary when considering male as when considering female sexual anatomy to remind ourselves of the importance of parts of the body other than the genitals, especially as many men appear to focus largely on their genitals during sexual behaviour. As a result, the very important non-genital aspects of the sex therapy programme (p. 128) can provide a novel and highly pleasurable experience for a man. However, in terms of specific knowledge required by the sex therapist, a full understanding of the anatomy of the male genitals is necessary.

External and internal genitals

The external genitals consist of the penis and scrotum (Fig. 2.4). The shaft of the penis contains three cylindrical bodies of erectile

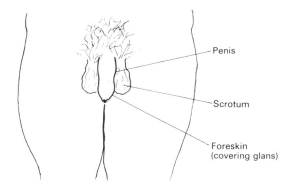

Fig. 2.4 Male external genitals

tissue—the two corpora cavernosa lying parallel to each other and above the corpus spongiosum, which contains the urethra (Fig. 2.5). The end of the corpus spongiosum forms the head of the penis, or glans. In the uncircumcized man this is covered by

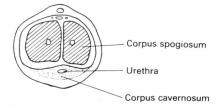

Fig. 2.5 Cross-section of the shaft of the penis

the retractable prepuce or foreskin. The glans is richly supplied with sensory nerve endings and is so sensitive that direct stimulation of the glans can be painful. The base of the glans is enlarged, forming the coronal ridge. Demarking the glans from the shaft of the penis is a groove, called the coronal sulcus. On the under-surface of the penis, between the glans and the shaft is a skin tag called the frenulum. The average length of the non-erect penis in most men is between 8.5 and 10.5 cm (3-4 in).

The scrotum is a sac of sensitive skin containing the testicles (Fig. 2.6). These are responsible for production of spermatozoa (in the seminiferous tubules of the testes) and sex hormones (from the Leydig cells lying in the interstitial tissue of the testes). Other internal genital structures are shown in Fig. 2.6. The prostate gland, which is approximately the size of a chestnut, lies below

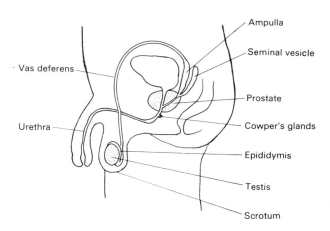

Fig. 2.6 Male internal genitals

the bladder. The urethra passes through it immediately after leaving the bladder. The prostate gland contributes some of the fluid to semen. The seminal vesicles produce most of the secretions contained in semen. The vas deferens is a tube-like structure that conveys spermatozoa from the testis to the prostatic urethra. Sperms are stored in the ampulla of the vas. A few drops of fluid may appear at the tip of the penis before ejaculation, and these are thought to be produced by Cowper's glands. However, the function of these glands is unknown.

MALE SEXUAL PHYSIOLOGY AND RESPONSE

The male sexual response cycle is shown schematically in Fig. 2.7. Some of the changes which occur during the various stages, including those involving parts of the body other than the genitals, are summarized in Table 2.2 at the end of this chapter. The response cycle may be divided into four stages in the same way as female sexual response. In addition, as in women, there is also the important factor of the background level of sexual interest, which will partly determine whether a man seeks out sexual opportunities and whether he responds to sexual advances.

Excitement phase

Erection of the penis is usually an early sign of sexual arousal. The mechanism of erection is unclear although a complicated

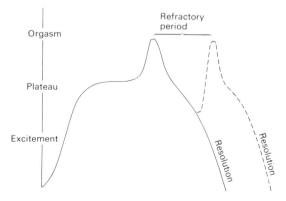

Fig. 2.7 Male sexual response

theoretical model which is supported by some experimental data has been proposed by Wagner (1981a). Essentially, it appears that erection depends on dilatation of the arterial vasculature of the penis, so that more blood enters the penis, and closure of venous valves, so that less blood flows out of the penis. The increase in size of the penis during erection is not directly proportional to the size of the flaccid organ. In fact, as Masters and Johnson (1966) were able to show, the increase in size of a small penis is often proportionately greater than that of a larger penis. The size of the erect penis for most men is in the range of 12.5-17.5 cm (5-7 in). The size and firmness of erection often fluctuates markedly during sexual arousal.

Plateau phase

During this stage of high sexual tension the penis undergoes further enlargement which is confined mostly to the coronal ridge of the glans penis. This phase varies in duration between individuals, and between different occasions in the same man. In men with premature ejaculation it is often extremely brief.

Orgasm

This is preceded in most men by a sense of 'ejaculatory inevitability' (sometimes called the 'point of no return'). It occurs when sexual tension increases to a point beyond which ejaculation is inevitable (the sexual response of some men with premature ejaculation is so rapid that they are unaware of this point). The sense of ejaculatory inevitability probably results from contraction of the accessory sex organs (prostate gland and seminal vesicles) causing emission of seminal fluid into the prostatic urethra. The second phase of ejaculation is expulsion of the seminal fluid along the length of the urethra and out of the urethral opening by rhythmic contraction of the prostate gland, perineal muscles, and shaft of the penis. During this stage the internal sphincter of the bladder is tightly closed to prevent the fluid passing backwards into the bladder.

Resolution

There is one important difference between this phase in men and the equivalent phase in the female sexual response cycle. Immediately after ejaculation there is a *refractory period* (Fig. 2.7) during which further ejaculation is impossible. This period varies from a few minutes to several hours or longer, and increases with age. Erection is lost in two stages; first, there is a rapid partial loss of erection, which is then followed by slower final detumescence.

Neurological basis of male sexual response

Apart from sensory nerve fibres supplying the skin of the external genitalia (carried in the pudendal nerve which leaves the sacral spinal cord at the levels S2-4), the main innervation of the penis subserving erection is two-fold. First, there is the parasympathetic nervous supply carried in the pelvic nerves which arise at levels S2-4 of the spinal cord, and, secondly, the sympathetic nervous supply carried in the hypogastric nerve which arises at levels T11-L3 of the cord. Parasympathetic and sympathetic nerves are involved in both the erectile response and ejaculation. Broadly speaking, parasympathetic activity is dominant during erection, and sympathetic activity dominant during ejaculation. The activity of these nerves is under the control of the brain. However, erection can also occur as a spinal reflex when higher control has been lost (e.g. following damage to the spinal cord).

Hormonal aspects of male sexual behaviour

The principal male sex hormones are androgens, namely *testosterone, dihydrotestosterone,* and *androstenedione.* Testosterone and androstenedione are mostly produced by the Leydig cells of the testes under the control of LH (luteinizing hormone). A small amount of androgen (especially dihydrotestosterone) is also produced by the adrenal cortex.

Testosterone appears to be important for maintaining sexual interest and the capacity for ejaculation. It is unclear whether it also has a direct role in the maintenance of erectile function, although hypogonadal men (i.e. with levels of circulating testosterone below the normal range) usually, but not always, experience some impairment of their erectile capacity (Davidson *et al.* 1982).

The effects of ageing on male sexuality

Peak levels of sexual arousability probably occur earlier in men than women, during the teens or early twenties. Later in life there does not seem to be the same precipitous hormonal change in men as occurs during the menopause in women. However, there is a gradual reduction in testosterone levels with increasing age. The main changes that occur with ageing are a decline in the length and intensity of the various phases of the sexual response cycle. An older man often takes longer and requires more stimulation in order to develop a full erection. The change in size of the penis during erection is less marked, and the firmness of erection is likely to be less than when he was younger. The angle of the erect penis (in relation to the abdomen) usually increases. More stimulation may be required before ejaculation occurs, ejaculation becomes less powerful, and the amount of semen produced is reduced. Also, the need to ejaculate seems to become less with increasing age. The resolution phase following ejaculation becomes more rapid. The refractory period may lengthen considerably, becoming several hours or even days long. As in women, other general effects of ageing, such as obesity, arthritis, illness, and medication, are also relevant to sexuality in older men.

However, older men often report considerable sexual satisfaction in spite of these changes and sexual activity is maintained by many men well into old age. For example, in Persson's (1980) study in Sweden, 46 per cent of 166 men aged 70 were found to be sexually active, the figure being 52 per cent for those who were married.

CONCLUSIONS

This chapter has included a brief description of the sexual anatomy and physiology of men and women, and the changes which occur during sexual response. Any therapist wishing to help people with sexual problems must have an adequate knowledge of sexual anatomy and sexual response. This will provide a basis for understanding sexual dysfunction. In addition, equipped with such knowledge, the therapist should be able to provide appropriate information which may facilitate treatment.

TABLE 2.1

Four-stage model of female sexual response (after Masters and Johnson 1966)

	Excitement	Plateau	Orgasm	Resolution
Vagina	Vaginal lubrication begins within 30 seconds of sexual stimulation; expansion and distension of inner ⅔ of vagina	Swelling of outer ⅓ of vagina ('orgasmic platform') leading to narrowing of vaginal entrance; further distension of inner ⅔ of vagina	Contractions (5-15) of outer ⅓ of vagina, gradually fading away	Disappearance of vaginal swelling and distension
Clitoris	Swelling of head of clitoris and elongation of shaft	Withdrawal of clitoral head and shaft into clitoral hood	No change	Rapid return to normal position; slower detumescence
Labia majora	Some separation (multipara) Increase in diameter (multipara)	Further engorgement	No reaction	Return to normal
Labia minora	Some thickening and expansion	Vivid colour change to deep red or wine colour	No reaction	Return to normal colour and size
Uterus	Elevation of body of uterus; cervix lifted from vaginal floor	Further elevation of body of uterus and of cervix	Uterine contractions from fundus of uterus to cervix	Return of uterus to normal position. Lowering of cervix to vaginal floor; gaping of cervical os

TABLE 2.1 (*cont.*)

	Excitement	Plateau	Orgasm	Resolution
Breasts	Nipple erection (not in all women, and may be delayed)	Breast enlargement; areolar engorgement	No change	Return to normal
General anatomical and physiological changes				
Skin	No reaction	'Sex flush', spreading from upper abdomen, over front of chest, neck, face, and forehead (not apparent in all women and varies from occasion to occasion)	'Sex flush' well developed	Rapid disappearance of 'sex flush'
Muscles	May be increase in muscle tension	Marked increase in muscle tension	Spasm of some muscle groups	Rapid relaxation
Pulse	Rate increases	Marked increase in rate	Maximal rate reached	Return to normal
Blood pressure	Some elevation	More marked elevation	Maximum level reached	Return to normal
Respiration	No change	Some increase in rate	Marked increase in rate	Return to normal

TABLE 2.2
Four-stage model of male sexual response (after Masters and Johnson 1966)

	Excitement	Plateau	Orgasm	Resolution
Penis	Rapid development of erection	Erection maintained; may be colour change of coronal ridge	Expulsive contractions of urethra, gradually fading away	Detumescence
Scrotum and testes	Thickening of scrotal skin; elevation of scrotum and testes	Enlargement and further elevation of testes	No reaction	Return to normal
Secondary organs (prostate, seminal vesicles, etc.)	No changes	No changes	Contraction, providing sensation of ejaculatory inevitability and causing emission of seminal fluid into prostatic urethra	No changes
Breasts	Nipple erection (some men)	Nipple erection (some men)	No changes	Return to normal
General anatomical and physiological changes				
Skin	No reaction	'Sex flush' (some men)	'Sex flush' well developed (some men)	Rapid disappearance of 'sex flush'
Muscles	May be increase in muscle tension	Marked increase in muscle tension	Spasm of some muscle groups	Rapid relaxation
Pulse	Rate increases	Marked increase in rate	Maximal rate reached	Return to normal
Blood pressure	Some elevation	More marked elevation	Maximum level reached	Return to normal
Respiration	No change	Some increase in rate	Marked increase in rate	Return to normal

Part I

Sexual problems

In this section various aspects of sexual dysfunction will be considered. Chapter 3 is largely devoted to description of the different types of sexual dysfunction. The ways in which sexual problems may present to helping agencies and the frequency with which the various types of dysfunction are seen in sexual dysfunction clinics will also be discussed. Chapter 4 summarizes the information currently available concerning the prevalence of sexual problems in the general population and in special clinical populations, and the deleterious effects that sexual problems may have on people's lives. The final chapter in this section is devoted to the causes of sexual problems, including a thorough examination of both psychological and physical causes, and the interaction between them. It provides an introduction to the rest of the book in which the management of sexual problems is described.

3

The nature of sexual problems

There is no universally accepted scheme for classifying the various types of sexual dysfunction, but recent approaches to classification have been far more sophisticated than in the past. At one time the terms 'frigidity' and 'impotence' were often used to indicate any sexual dysfunction of women and men respectively. Both are non-specific and are often used perjoratively. In addition, 'frigidity' suggests, usually incorrectly, an association with lack of emotional warmth. This term should be avoided. The word 'impotence' has been used more specifically, as in 'erectile impotence'. However, as erectile difficulty is often not complete, and given the somewhat pejorative overtones of the word 'impotent', the descriptive term 'erectile dysfunction' is preferable and will be used in this book.

Masters and Johnson (1970) classified sexual problems of women into three categories: orgasmic dysfunction, vaginismus, and dyspareunia. Those of men were classified into four categories: impotence, premature ejaculation, ejaculatory incompetence, and dyspareunia. On the basis of her biphasic concept of sexual response (p. 7), Kaplan (1974) proposed a classification system in which disorders of sexual arousal (general sexual dysfunction in women, and erectile dysfunction or impotence in men) were distinguished from disorders of orgasm (orgasmic dysfunction in women, and premature ejaculation and retarded ejaculation in men). In addition, Kaplan recognized that vaginismus had to be considered separately from the two components of her biphasic scheme.

During the 1970s it became apparent to therapists that many couples seeking help had problems other than those of sexual arousal and orgasm. In particular, many women had problems concerning their level of sexual interest or desire. In 1977, Kaplan modified her biphasic concept of sexual response, introducing a triphasic model in which she distinguished *sexual desire* from *excitement* (or arousal) and *orgasm*. She emphasized that 'hypoactive sexual desire' was a common complaint among both women and men who sought help, and that, in many cases, it seemed to be a complicated problem requiring extensive therapy, often going beyond the usual sex therapy format (Kaplan 1979). In the author's clinical practice, a classification system similar to Kaplan's has been found useful, and this is the system of classification which will be described here. It differs from Kaplan's mainly with regard to the terms used.

In addition to specific dysfunctions it is extremely important to take account of another dimension of human sexuality, namely *sexual satisfaction*. A person's satisfaction with a sexual relationship may not depend just on the presence or absence of sexual dysfunction, but on other aspects of the relationship, both sexual and non-sexual (Frank *et al.* 1976; Chesney *et al.* 1981; Perlman and Abramson 1982). This important dimension of sexuality must also be included in any description of sexual problems and is discussed further below.

A working definition of sexual dysfunction is *the persistent impairment of the normal patterns of sexual interest or response*. As with most attempts at defining broad categories of personal problems, this definition is open to considerable criticism. For example, the word 'normal' raises the issue of what should be regarded as normal in human sexuality when the range of sexual interest and performance is so broad, both in the same individual at various times and between different individuals. Secondly, it could be argued quite reasonably that judgement concerning whether or not a person has a sexual dysfunction requiring treatment should depend on whether the person perceives himself or herself as having a sexual problem, and also whether the person's partner thinks there is a problem.

The classification system that will now be described has proved satisfactory in working with people with sexual problems. It has the advantage that it accommodates nearly all the patients with sexual dysfunction that are seen in clinical practice. The types of dysfunction of women and men are listed in Table 3.1. They are grouped in four categories, namely those of problems affecting *sexual interest, arousal* and *orgasm,* and *other problems* which cannot be included in the first three categories.

Two further important dimensions of classification, which were recognized by Masters and Johnson (1970), are the time of onset of a problem and the situations in which it occurs. First, a dysfunction may be either primary or secondary. A *primary dysfunction* is one that has been experienced continuously by a person since sexual activity first began. A *secondary dysfunction* is one which has arisen after a period of satisfactory sexual functioning. Any dysfunction can be either primary or secondary, although there is some variation in the extent to which particular problems are more often primary or secondary. For example, vaginismus is usually a primary problem, whereas erectile dysfunction is more commonly a secondary problem. Secondly, Masters and Johnson (1970) also suggested the term *situational* to describe a problem which occurs in one setting and not in another, and *total* for problems which occur in all settings. For example, a man who cannot obtain an erection when with a partner but can have a good erection on his own has a situational problem, as does a woman who is unable to have an orgasm with her current partner, but can on her own or with another partner. A *total* problem would occur in all such sexual situations.

THE SEXUAL PROBLEMS OF WOMEN

Impaired sexual interest

This is the most common problem among women seen in sexual dysfunction clinics. As with other types of dysfunction, this diagnostic category includes a wide range of difficulties. Thus, some women lack spontaneous interest in sex but are able to respond to their partners' approaches and experience arousal and orgasm, while others may both lack interest in initiating sexual activity and be averse to the sexual approaches of their partners.

TABLE 3.1
Classification of the sexual dysfunctions of women and men

Aspects of sexuality affected	Sexual dysfunction	
	Women	*Men*
Sexual interest	Impaired sexual interest	Impaired sexual interest
Arousal	Impaired sexual arousal	Erectile dysfunction
Orgasm	Orgasmic dysfunction	Premature ejaculation Retarded ejaculation Ejaculatory pain
Other types of dysfunction	Vaginismus Dyspareunia Sexual phobias	Dyspareunia Sexual phobias

In evaluating whether a woman has a problem concerning her level of sexual interest one must take into account, first, the wide range of sexual interest among women in the general population, secondly, the woman's previous level of sexual interest, and thirdly, her expectations and whether or not she thinks she has a problem. In assessing a woman's level of sexual interest she should be asked not only about the extent to which she feels interested in having sex with her partner, but also about her frequency of spontaneous sexual thoughts and fantasies, frequency of masturbation, and whether she feels attracted to other men. This will help to clarify whether her impaired sexual interest is situational (e.g. partner-related) or total.

In women with primary impairment of sexual interest, negative experiences relatively early in life are likely to be important causal factors, whereas in those with secondary impairment of sexual interest, who form a larger group among clients of sexual dysfunction clinics, the problem is often associated with difficulties in a woman's general relationship with her partner, or follows a clear precipitant such as childbirth or depression (see Chapter 5).

Impaired sexual arousal

Problems of sexual arousal are characterized by failure of the physiological responses which normally occur during this phase (p. 12), especially vaginal swelling and lubrication, and by lack of the sensations usually associated with sexual excitement. Such problems are relatively uncommon in women with unimpaired sexual interest. However, after childbirth and following the menopause, hormonal changes may impair the normal vaginal response to sexual stimulation.

Orgasmic dysfunction

It has already been noted that enjoyment of sexual activity without reaching orgasm does not necessarily constitute a problem (p. 14); the extent to which a woman regards herself as having a problem concerning orgasm will in part depend on her expectations. These may change with time and because of information in the media; sometimes such information can set up unreasonable expectations (p. 65).

When deciding which treatment approach is most appropriate it is important to establish whether a woman's orgasmic dysfunction is total (i.e. orgasm is never experienced during sexual activity of any kind) or situational (i.e. orgasm occurs under some circumstances (most likely masturbation) but not others). Primary total orgasmic dysfunction is relatively common, although some sex therapists have noticed a recent reduction in the numbers of women presenting for help with this problem. This might be the result of articles in popular journals concerning masturbation and self-help programmes, as well as publication of self-help books (e.g. Barbach 1976; Heiman *et al.* 1976). Secondary orgasmic dysfunction is often related to difficulties in a woman's general relationship with her partner (McGovern *et al.* 1975). It may also be associated with secondary impairment of sexual interest, in which case the latter is usually the main problem and should be the focus of treatment.

Vaginismus

In this condition, sexual intercourse is either impossible or extremely painful because spasm of the muscles surrounding the entrance to the vagina occurs when penetration is attempted. The spasm is an automatic response over which the woman feels she has no control. This is a major cause of non-consummation of marriage. It may also occur as a mild transient problem when a woman first starts having sexual intercourse. Vaginismus is usually a primary dysfunction. However, it may develop as a secondary problem following vaginal trauma, such as a poorly repaired episiotomy, or recurrent vaginal infections, when vaginal penetration may be painful. Eventually, anticipation of pain can lead to spasm of the perineal muscles whenever penetration is attempted.

In most cases of vaginismus there is a specific phobia concerning vaginal penetration. Careful enquiry will often elicit a history of difficult first attempts at insertion of tampons which the woman was never subsequently able to use. Women with vaginismus occasionally have extreme fears about childbirth. It is quite common to find that the woman has distorted ideas about her genitals, usually thinking that her vagina is far too small to accommodate a penis. Her partner may collude with this belief. In some cases the woman also regards her genitals as unclean or unpleasant in some other way. One patient said she thought her vagina was like an open wound. Such distorted ideas are usually maintained because the woman never attempts to examine herself, either visually or with her fingers. However, primary vaginismus occasionally has a physical basis, such as a tough unruptured hymen.

Many women with vaginismus resulting from a specific phobia about penetration are sexually responsive. In a series of 30 women presenting for help for this condition, 56 per cent had achieved orgasm through petting, 41 per cent in dreams, and 28 per cent through masturbation (Duddle 1977). The proportion experiencing orgasm through petting and dreams was in excess of that of a control group of women seeking contraceptive advice in a family planning clinic, and the proportion who masturbated to orgasm was the same as in the comparison group.

Vaginismus is sometimes part of a more extensive sexual disorder, in which there is general inhibition of sexual interest, and often aversion to sexual contact. In contrast with the more usual type of vaginismus, such cases can be difficult to treat; the general sexual difficulties must be the initial focus of therapy before any attempt is made to help the woman accept vaginal penetration.

Dyspareunia

This refers to pain during sexual intercourse. Sometimes coital pain is localized at the entrance to the vagina, in which case it may be the result of one of several factors, including mild vaginismus, lack of arousal, a vaginal infection, or a Bartholin's cyst. Pain resulting from lack of arousal usually eases as sexual intercourse proceeds because vaginal lubrication increases and the vaginal muscles relax. Dyspareunia on deep penetration often has a physical basis (e.g. vaginal infection, such as 'thrush' or herpes, pelvic infection, ovarian pathology, or endometriosis). The pain becomes worse with thrusting and usually does not diminish during sexual intercourse. However, sometimes deep dyspareunia results from impaired sexual arousal, when ballooning of the inner part of the vagina and elevation of the uterus (Table 2.1) do not occur. The cervix is thus subject to intense buffeting by the penis which causes the woman pain and may therefore lead to further inhibition of her arousal. It is most important that a physical cause of dyspareunia is always suspected until ruled out by detailed assessment and a gynaecological examination.

Sexual phobias

These may occur as an isolated problem, or, more commonly, in association with other dysfunctions, such as impaired sexual interest or arousal. The phobia may be very specific, such as aversion to touching the partner's penis or to seminal fluid, or more generalized, such as aversion to foreplay. A sexual phobia need not necessarily prevent a woman from enjoying the rest of sexual activity, but in some cases the phobia completely inhibits sexual arousal. Sexual phobias are occasionally related to an earlier traumatic experience, such as rape or incest.

THE SEXUAL PROBLEMS OF MEN

Impaired sexual interest

Although all men, as well as women, occasionally lose interest in sex, it is relatively rare for men to seek help specifically for this problem. One reason may be that reduced sexual interest often causes a disorder of sexual performance, such as erectile dysfunction, and it is for this problem that the man is more likely to seek help. Another possible reason stems from the myth that men are always ready and able to have sex; this might make it difficult for many men to acknowledge that their desire for sex is absent or reduced. Couples occasionally seek help because the man's level of sexual interest is less than that of the partner.

When impaired interest in sex is a primary problem, a careful check must be made for a possible organic cause, such as an endocrine disturbance (e.g. hypogonadism). As in women, secondary impaired interest in sex in men is often the result of disturbance in the general relationship with the partner, although depression and physical illness are other common causes.

Erectile dysfunction

This is the most common sexual dysfunction among men who seek help for causal problems. Such men are on average older than those presenting with other dysfunctions, especially ejaculatory disorders. The erectile response is very vulnerable to psychological influences, particularly anxiety, and to physical disorders and side-effects of drugs, including alcohol (Chapter 5).

The range of erectile disorders is considerable. Primary, total erectile dysfunction is relatively rare, and usually has a physical basis. When this form of erectile disorder is incomplete, that is the man can obtain partial erections, a physical cause is again likely. Sometimes a disorder of the blood supply of the penis, such as leakage from the penile cavernous bodies, can result in a man never being able to get more than a partial erection (Wagner and Green 1981). Primary situational erectile dysfunction, which normally means a man can obtain erections on his own but not with a partner, or cannot sustain his erection when sexual intercourse is attempted, usually has a psychological basis.

Premature ejaculation

There is no entirely satisfactory definition of premature ejaculation. Rapid ejaculation is common in young men having their first sexual encounters. Subsequently, most men will develop some control over their speed of ejaculation during sexual inter-course. Masters and Johnson (1970) defined premature ejaculation in terms of the extent to which a man could delay ejaculation long enough during sexual intercourse for his partner to reach orgasm. This is obviously unsatisfactory, because the partner may herself have a problem in responding which may be uncon-nected with the man's ejaculatory control. Clearly, ejaculation which occurs before vaginal penetration, or immediately after penetration, is premature. The best guide as to whether there really is a problem in milder cases is the extent to which the couple feel that the man's ejaculatory control is sufficient to allow intercourse which is satisfactory for them both. At this point it is worth noting Kinsey and colleagues' (1948) finding that three-quarters of the married men they interviewed estimated that they ejaculated within two minutes of vaginal penetration. These authors unfortunately did not report how many of the men regarded this as a problem.

Premature ejaculation is usually a primary problem. There is often a history of rapid masturbation, sometimes associated with feelings of guilt. This might predispose to premature ejaculation when a man establishes a sexual relationship. The partner's reaction to his rapid ejaculation may be crucial; if this is one of anger and condemnation, loss of confidence may cause even more rapid ejaculation. Many men with premature ejaculation try using distracting thoughts during sexual intercourse, which only reduces the pleasure of the act, or anaesthetic creams, which are equally helpful. Often a couple shorten their foreplay in the hope that this will help, although usually it does not. It is not surprising that premature ejaculation is commonly associated with orgasmic dysfunction or impaired sexual interest in the partner (p. 65). Young men with only a brief refractory period following a first ejaculation often compensate for premature ejaculation by being able to sustain sexual intercourse longer before ejaculating a second time. However, as the refractory period lengthens with ageing (p. 22) premature ejaculation may then become a problem.

Premature ejaculation sometimes develops as a secondary problem at a time of stress. It also often occurs transiently when a man's frequency of sexual intercourse has been reduced for some reason, such as absence from his partner. However, premature ejaculation sometimes precedes erectile dysfunction caused by either psychological or physical factors.

Retarded ejaculation

This disorder, which affects both ejaculation and the experience of orgasm, is relatively uncommon. It includes a range of problems, such as total failure of ejaculation under any circumstances (including masturbation and sleep), partial failure, when ejaculation is not possible with a partner but does occur in masturbation, and difficulty in ejaculating, when sexual stimulation or intercourse must be continued for an excessively long time for ejaculation to occur. Several forms of medication can also interfere with ejaculation (Table 5.5). Some men with this problem are thought to be over-controlled individuals who resist 'letting themselves go' because of hostile feelings towards their partners (Kaplan 1974). However, total failure of ejaculation is likely to have a physical basis.

Failure of ejaculation must be distinguished from *retrograde ejaculation*, in which a man has the subjective experience of orgasm but does not produce any ejaculate from his penis. This condition is usually caused by physical factors (e.g. prostatectomy, diabetes, major tranquillizers) which inhibit the action of the internal sphincter of the bladder, thus allowing the ejaculate to pass back into the bladder. Following orgasm the man may notice that his urine is cloudy because it contains seminal fluid.

Ejaculatory pain and dyspareunia

These conditions are uncommon. Painful ejaculation is usually associated with infection involving the urethra, seminal vesicles, prostate gland, or bladder. Often the complaint is of a burning sensation in the penis after ejaculation. Some perfectly healthy men experience hyperaesthesia of the glans penis after ejaculation so that the glans is very painful if touched. Kaplan (1979) has also suggested that painful ejaculation and post-ejaculatory pain may occasionally be caused by spasm of the perineal muscles because of a man's anxiety about ejaculation.

Pain during sexual intercourse usually suggests a physical cause, such as a tight foreskin, local infection, or a tear of the frenulum.

Sexual phobias

Men rarely present for help because of aversion to specific aspects of sexual behaviour. However, a phobia may be an important component of another dysfunction. For example, some men with erectile dysfunction experience aversion to extreme sexual excitement in their partners, or to vaginal lubrication.

SEXUAL DISSATISFACTION

So far we have concentrated on sexual dysfunctions. However, as noted earlier in this chapter, another important dimension of sexuality is sexual satisfaction; that is, the extent to which a person is content with, and enjoys his or her sexual relationship. Although sexual satisfaction often accompanies sexual dysfunction this is not always so. In a study of 100 married couples who volunteered for interview, Frank and colleagues (1978) found that sexual dissatisfaction correlated only weakly with the presence of sexual dysfunction in the wives, and not at all in the men. Sexual dissatisfaction was more strongly associated with 'sexual difficulties' (e.g. 'difficulty relaxing', 'too little foreplay') than with sexual dysfunction. However, most couples who present to sexual dysfunction clinics are dissatisfied with their sexual relationship (Frank *et al.* 1976). Some specifically complain of 'lack of enjoyment', although this is often secondary to impaired sexual interest (Bancroft 1983).

Many other factors may contribute to sexual dissatisfaction. It often reflects difficulties in the general relationship between partners. Thus, a dysfunction might be tolerated by many couples if their relationship is otherwise happy; they might also stand a better chance of solving the problem without outside help (Chesney *et al.* 1981). Further factors include loss of attraction between partners and lack of variation or experimentation in sexual activity.

PRESENTATION OF SEXUAL PROBLEMS

How help for sexual problems is sought

Some people approach their family doctors with *direct requests* for help with sexual difficulties. With increasing publicity about sexual problems and sex therapy it appears that more people are now willing to make such a direct approach for help. Others, however, may be too embarrassed to express their concerns directly, or may not even realize that there is a sexual cause for the difficulty they are experiencing, and therefore they present for help *indirectly*. Whether or not the true nature of the problem is detected, and how long this takes, will depend on their doctors' awareness of sexual problems and their presentation, and, in particular, their willingness to inquire about this area of patient's lives. Indirect presentations may come in the guise of emotional or psychological problems (such as depression, marital disharmony, insomnia), or gynaecological complaints (such as requests for a change of contraceptive pill, or repeated concern about normal vaginal discharge). Sexual problems may also present indirectly in gynaecology clinics, psychiatry out-patients, and infertility clinics. For example, it is not uncommon for couples who are unable to have satisfactory sexual intercourse because of vaginismus, erectile dysfunction, or failure of ejaculation, to present initially to an infertility clinic. Couples occasionally request help because they have unrealistically high expectations of their sexual relationships.

Sources of referrals for sex therapy

To some extent the sources of referrals to a sexual dysfunction clinic will depend on the setting of the clinic and the links that it has with other health care settings. The author has been involved in a sexual dysfunction clinic in a psychiatric setting. During a seven-year period 794 referrals were received. The majority (60 per cent) came from family doctors, 16 per cent from other psychiatrists, 9 per cent from gynaecologists and 16 per cent from a variety of other sources including physicians and venereology and family planning clinics. The fact that all referrals passed via medical agencies is the result of the policy of the clinic to ensure as far as possible that people who require physical attention for their sexual difficulties have been screened out. However, referrals of cases in which sexual dysfunction is the result of psychological reactions to a physical disorder are encouraged.

Frequency of presentation of different types of sexual dysfunction

Several reports are now available concerning the patterns of sexual problems seen in sexual dysfunction clinics. Differences in diagnostic practices mean unfortunately that direct comparison between clinics is not always possible. The pattern of referrals to the author's clinic during a seven-year period are summarized in Table 3.2.

TABLE 3.2

Frequency of different types of sexual problems among men and women presenting to a sexual dysfunction clinic

Women (N = 257)	%
Impaired sexual interest	52
Orgasmic dysfunction	19
Vaginismus	18
Dyspareunia	4
Other	7

Men (N = 258)	%
Erectile dysfunction	60
Premature ejaculation	16
Retarded ejaculation	6
Impaired sexual interest	6
Other	12

Most of the referrals were of couples. In each case only the sexual problem of the presenting partner is recorded.

The frequency of referral of the various types of sexual dysfunctions is similar to that reported from elsewhere, including the same clinic during an earlier three-year period (Bancroft and Coles 1976), a family planning centre (Duddle 1975), psychiatry clinics (Cooper 1979), and two other sexual dysfunction clinics (Milne, 1976; Bancroft 1983). Couples presenting with sexual problems to Marriage Guidance differed in that orgasmic dysfunction and premature ejaculation were encountered more often in that setting (Heisler 1983).

Broadly speaking, the proportions of couples in which the women or the men are the presenting partners are similar. The average age of the men is greater than that of the women because of a subgroup of older men among those with erectile dysfunction. Impaired sexual interest in women and erectile dysfunction are the most common presenting problems.

Often an individual has more than one sexual problem. In women, orgasmic dysfunction is commonly found in association with impaired sexual interest, and in men, premature ejaculation is often linked with erectile dysfunction. In addition, in many couples both partners have sexual problems. Various estimates have been made of the proportion of couples attending sexual dysfunction clinics in whom this is so, and these have ranged from 25 per cent (Kaplan 1974), through 30 per cent (Bancroft 1983), 36 per cent (Hawton 1982), and 44 per cent (Masters and Johnson 1970), to 48 per cent (Crowe *et al.* 1981). The most common association is between impaired sexual interest in the woman and premature ejaculation in her partner (Hawton 1982). Very often the two problems are interrelated, with one being exacerbated or caused by the other.

CONCLUSIONS

In this chapter the nature and presentation of sexual problems of men and women have been examined. A classification scheme that is currently found useful in clinical practice has been described. People do not always present with direct requests for help for their sexual difficulties. Often they initially seek help for other psychological or physical complaints. Identification of the true nature of their problems may depend on the skill and attitudes of the person who assesses them. Sexual dysfunction in a couple is often not confined to the presenting partner; in approximately a third of cases both partners have sexual difficulties, the problems of each commonly being interrelated.

4

The prevalence and effects
of sexual problems

When considering the need for treatment facilities for people
with sexual problems, two initial questions must be answered.
First, how many people experience sexual problems? Secondly,
what effects do sexual difficulties have on people's lives and
relationships? A further question concerns the effectiveness of
treatment methods, but this is more appropriately considered
separately (see Chapters 13 and 14). This chapter will address
the first two questions in some detail.

THE PREVALENCE OF SEXUAL PROBLEMS

Surveys designed to determine the frequency of sexual problems
in a population encounter many methodological difficulties. These
should be taken into account when assessing such findings, and
include the following:

1. *Sample selection.* Usually it is not feasible to survey all the
members of a population; the method by which the sample for
survey is selected is therefore crucial. Ideally the sample should
be selected on a random basis and be of sufficient size to minimize
the likelihood of misleading chance findings.

2. *Response rate.* Not all the people who are approached for
inclusion in a survey will give their consent; refusals are probably

more likely when the survey concerns sexuality. Non-responders may differ in important ways from those who agree to their inclusion. Therefore, even a small non-response rate might cause quite marked distortions of the findings of a survey.

3. *How questions are asked.* Broadly speaking, there are two methods of survey, the first by questionnaire, and the second by personal interview. The two approaches are likely to produce different results. Survey by questionnaire removes the risks of bias in response that might be introduced by an interviewer; if completed anonymously, a questionnaire might, arguably, also elicit more honest and accurate responses. On the other hand, survey by interview allows much greater depth of questioning, but risks the interviewer's own source of bias unless the interviews are carefully standardized and their reliability checked.

4. *Validity of responses.* Because of the embarrassment and defensiveness that many people show when asked about their sexuality, and the pressure thay may feel to match up to 'expected standards', doubt often surrounds the accuracy of elicited information. Answers may be corroborated to some degree by asking similar questions of a sexual partner.

5. *Definitions of sexual problems.* As we have already noted, at present there is no universally accepted scheme for classifying sexual problems. It is often very difficult, therefore, to compare findings from different surveys. Moreover, surveys in which sexual problems have not been defined operationally provide findings which are difficult to interpret.

6. *Resistance to surveys.* A final problem is the resistance shown by many people, including fellow professionals, to surveys concerning sexuality.

Given all these difficulties, it is not surprising that few surveys of the prevalence of sexual difficulties in defined populations have been carried out, and that most of these are heavily flawed.

In examining the evidence concerning the prevalence of sexual problems we shall begin by considering studies of sexual difficulties in the general population. Then, because of the recognized association of sexual problems with many physical and psychiatric disorders (Chapter 5), we shall turn our attention to studies of patients in clinical settings, where sexual difficulties are likely to be detected because people come under special scrutiny.

General population surveys

When setting up a clinical service for people with sexual difficulties, three factors are likely to affect the demand for treatment: first, the frequency with which sexual problems exist in the general population; secondly, the extent to which people with problems wish for help; and thirdly, the extent to which such people are detected or seek help themselves, and, when appropriate, are referred to a specialized service. Where individuals are able directly to approach a specialized helping agency, such as Marriage Guidance, then the demand will partly also depend on how well such an agency advertises itself. Here we will consider the first two factors, namely the prevalence of sexual problems in the general population and the extent to which people wish for help with them.

The first and most extensive general population surveys of sexuality were those of Kinsey and his colleagues (1948, 1953). Between 1938 and the late 1940s this research team carried out very detailed interviews with more than 6000 men and almost 6000 women in the USA. Although the surveys were in many respects based on rigorous scientific principles, unfortunately the sample of subjects who were interviewed was not representative of the general population of the country. There was a marked bias towards higher educational status, and many of the subjects were obtained through personal contact, while others were identified through social and work organizations. Nevertheless, the surveys have provided us with a very rich source of information concerning sexuality of men and women during the first half of this century. It is quite difficult to draw from the findings data relevant to the question of how many individuals experienced sexual dysfunction, but the following statistics are probably the most important.

Among the *men* (Kinsey *et al.* 1948), the prevalence of 'more or less total impotence' increased exponentially with age: 0.1 per cent at age 20, 0.8 per cent at age 30, 1.9 per cent at age 40, 6.7 per cent at age 50, 18.4 per cent at age 60, 27 per cent at age 70, and over 50 per cent for men aged 75 or more. Some workers from the Kinsey Institute have subsequently provided more refined data from the Kinsey survey (Gebhard and Johnson 1979). They reported that 5.6 per cent of white college-educated men and 18.9 per cent of white non-college-educated men experienced regular erectile dysfunction when attempting sexual intercourse. Although the Kinsey study did not ascertain the prevalence of premature ejaculation, it did provide data relevant to this problem. For example, 3.8 per cent of men said that during sexual intercourse they ejaculated within one minute of penetration (based on Gebhard and Johnsons' (1979) recalculation of the original data). We do not know what proportion of these men felt that ejaculation was out of their control or regarded their speed of ejaculation as a problem. Kinsey and colleagues reported that failure of ejaculation was a very rare phenomenon, occurring in only 6 out of 4108 men. Their survey provided no information concerning disorders of sexual interest in men.

In the survey of *women* (Kinsey *et al.* 1953), there is much data concerning orgasm but again none concerning sexual interest. Among married women the proportion who never experienced orgasm decreased steadily with age, being 22 per cent among those aged 16-20, 12 per cent in those aged 21-25, and 5-7 per cent in those aged between 30 and 50. Overall, almost 13 per cent of married women had never experienced orgasm through any means (Gebhard and Johnson 1979).

More recent information concerning the prevalence of sexual problems has been provided by Frank and her colleagues in the USA (1978). They gave a self-report questionnaire concerning many aspects of marriage to 100 couples recruited from a variety of sources, including clubs and church groups. Only couples who 'believed their marriages were working' were asked to volunteer. The sample is in no sense random. It was largely middle-class, and participation rates ranged from only 5 to 50 per cent of couples in different groups who were approached. The investigators distinguished between 'dysfunctions' (erectile and ejaculatory problems in the husbands, and arousal and orgasmic problems in the wives), and 'difficulties' (e.g. 'too little foreplay before intercourse', 'inability to relax', and 'attraction to person(s) other than the mate'.). Among the wives, 63 per cent reported one or more sexual dysfunction, of which 'difficulty getting excited' (48 per cent) and 'difficulty in reaching orgasm' (46 per cent) were the most common. Fifteen per cent said they were unable to have an orgasm at all. Of the husbands, 40 per cent admitted to one or more sexual dysfunction, of which premature ejaculation (36 per cent) was the most common. Difficulty in getting an erection was reported by 7 per cent and difficulty maintaining an erection by 9 per cent. Four per cent had difficulty in ejaculating.

Sexual difficulties were reported more frequently than sexual dysfunctions, namely by 77 per cent of the wives and 50 per cent of the husbands. The main difficulties cited were, by the wives, 'inability to relax', 'too little foreplay before intercourse', and 'disinterest', and, by the men, 'attraction to person(s) other than the mate', and 'too little foreplay before intercourse'. 'Disinterest' was reported by 35 per cent of the wives and 16 per cent of the husbands.

In spite of the limitations of this study, it produced some findings of particular interest. For example, there was a marked sex difference in the perception of the partners' sexual problems. While the wives were well aware of the dysfunctions reported by their husbands, many of the men failed to recognize the problems experienced by their wives. In addition, sexual dissatisfaction was more strongly correlated with sexual difficulties than with dysfunction. Indeed in men there was no obvious association between sexual dysfunction and dissatisfaction. Among the wives, 'difficulty getting excited' was the dysfunction most strongly correlated with dissatisfaction, although there was a small correlation between dissatisfaction and orgasmic difficulties.

In a personal interview survey of a random sample of 225 40-year old Danish women, Garde and Lunde (1980a) found that 35 per cent reported current sexual problems. These were combinations of the dysfunctions and difficulties identified by Frank and colleagues. It is unfortunate that the problems were not defined more clearly. The most common problem was 'too little motivation' (42 per cent of those with problems), which presumably means lack of sexual interest. Other sexual problems included 'derives nothing from intercourse' (20 per cent), 'feels it is an obligation' (16.5 per cent), and 'partner derives nothing from intercourse' (6 per cent). Although virtually all the women had experienced orgasm at some time in their lives, two-thirds reported having simulated orgasm. A third of the women said they had never experienced 'spontaneous sexual desire', and 12 per cent had not experienced 'libido' under any circumstances. Sexual problems were far more common among lower-social-class women than those of higher social class (Garde and Lunde 1980b). Almost a third of the women with problems wished to obtain advice, although many were pessimistic about whether they could be helped.

Sexual dysfunction and sexual satisfaction were studied in 58 Swedish married men by Nettelbladt and Uddenberg (1979). The men were identified as part of a broader study of randomly selected Swedish families and were interviewed using a semi-structured questionnaire. A 'tendency towards sexual dysfunction' was reported by 40 per cent of the men. Premature ejaculation was experienced by 38 per cent of the sample, a proportion almost identical to that found by Frank and colleagues. This was defined as 'failure to control ejaculation and therefore reaching orgasm too fast on at least a third of occasions of sexual intercourse'. Interestingly, 10 per cent of the men reported retarded ejaculation. Erectile dysfunction (failure to get an erection sufficient for vaginal penetration on at least 50 per cent of occasions) occurred in 7 per cent. This figure is also very similar to that reported by Frank and colleagues. Again, as in the study by the American group, reported satisfaction with the sexual relationship was not related to sexual dysfunction in these Swedish men. This perhaps reflects the rather wide definitions of sexual dysfunctions, for as the authors suggest, 'occasional sexual dysfunction may not interfere with sexual satisfaction'. Nevertheless, the similarities between the findings of the two studies are remarkable.

Some other general population surveys of sexuality and sexual difficulties have had little or no scientific basis but three are worth noting in passing. The first was a survey in 1974 of women readers of *Redbook Magazine* in the USA (Tavris and Sadd 1977). Over 100 000 married women completed and returned a questionnaire about sexuality which was published in the magazine. Clearly the sample was not representative of the general population of married women; in addition to having a middle-class bias, the group of women who responded to the questionnaire were unlikely to have been representative of the married female readership of the magazine. Nevertheless, the following findings are of interest. Seven per cent of women never reached orgasm in sexual intercourse, and 11 per cent reported that coital orgasm occurred 'once in a while' (15 per cent reported they always reach orgasm in intercourse). Thirty eight per cent said that sexual intercourse occurred 'too infrequently'. In response to the question 'In general, how would you evaluate the sexual aspect of your marriage?', 12 per cent said it was 'poor' or 'very poor'. The percentages of women who gave such a response increased steadily the longer they had been married.

Hite (1976) collected the replies of more than 3000 women in the USA to a questionnaire concerning sexuality. The sample was obtained through personal contact, advertisements in magazines, and women's organizations. Apart from the obvious sources of bias that must occur in a survey of this kind, the response rate was very low with only just over 3000 completed questionnaires returned out of 100 000 that were sent out. A complete absence of orgasm was reported by almost 12 per cent of women. Orgasm was 'rarely' (or never) achieved during sexual intercourse by 17 per cent of women. As in some of the other surveys, no questions relevant to levels of sexual interest were asked.

Finally, mention should be made of Fisher's (1973) study of a small and highly selected group of American women, most of whom were attending college. Between 5 and 6 per cent of the women had never experienced orgasm.

We can only reach tentative conclusions when trying to draw together the findings of these general population surveys. First, it is clear that sexual problems are not rare. Secondly, it appears that sexual problems are more common among women than men, or at least that women more often admit to sexual difficulties. There may also be a greater incidence among those of lower social class. Thirdly, the prevalence of sexual dysfunction in women is probably between 35 and 60 per cent, with impaired sexual interest and arousability being the most common. Complete failure to reach orgasm is found in between 10 and 15 per cent of married women. No information is available concerning the prevalence of vaginismus. Finally, although the incidence of male sexual dysfunction is less clear, partly because men have rarely been surveyed, the studies of married men by Frank and colleagues (1978) and by Nettelbladt and Uddenberg (1979) were in remarkable agreement in suggesting that 40 per cent of such men have some degree of dysfunction. Premature ejaculation seems to be the most common problem, being found in 20-40 per cent of married men. Erectile dysfunction occurs in 7-10 per cent, the incidence increasing with age. Retarded ejaculation is less common, occurring probably at most in 4 per cent of married men. Clearly, not everyone identified as having a sexual dysfunction will see it as a problem. Thus there appears to be a poor correlation between the presence of sexual dysfunction and sexual satisfaction, especially in men. Many other factors will influence this, including, in particular, the general emotional atmosphere of a relationship (p. 70). Even when a problem is recognized, a person may not wish for help with it. For example, a third of the women with sexual problems in the study by Garde and Lunde (1980a) actually wanted help. However, this still represents a substantial number of individuals. The great demand for treatment that became apparent when sexual dysfunction clinics were first established (Bancroft and Coles 1976), and which has continued ever since (Hawton 1982), has provided clear practical evidence that many people are troubled by their sexual difficulties and want help.

Surveys of patients in clinical settings

Burnap and Golden (1967) interviewed *physicians in a variety of specialities* in the USA to survey retrospectively the frequency with which they saw patients with sexual difficulties. The highest frequencies, apart from those obtained from psychiatrists, were reported by doctors in general practice, urology, and obstetrics and gynaecology, who thought that an average of 15 per cent of their patients had sexual problems. The most frequent types of sexual problems reported were 'lack of orgasm during intercourse', 'frigidity, or lack of desire for intercourse', 'lack of sexual information, no specific problem', and 'impotence or lack of erection during intercourse'. It is of interest that Burnap and Golden reported that the frequencies with which sexual problems were apparently encountered by the physicians were more closely related to the characteristics of the physicians themselves than to those of their patients. The relevant characteristics of the physicians were, first, whether they routinely asked about sex problems, and secondly, whether they appeared uncomfortable when talking about sexuality with the research interviewers. Those who were more uncomfortable (blushing, excessive joking, suspicious, resentful) reported much lower frequencies of sexual problems in their patients than those who appeared more comfortable with the topic.

The family planning clinic is an obvious setting in which sexual difficulties might easily be identified. Begg *et al.* (1976) surveyed by questionnaire 759 consecutive women who attended a large family planning clinic in Edinburgh during one week. These constituted a predominantly young population (75 per cent less than 30 years old) with a large proportion of unmarried subjects (40 per cent). More than 90 per cent of those approached completed the questionnaire, and 12.5 per cent indicated that they 'had a sexual problem at the present time'. Of these, more than three-quarters said they wanted help for the problem. Overall, 9.5 per cent of women indicated that they had a sexual problem and wanted help for it. The women's partners (if they attended) were also asked to complete questionnaires; only 5.7 per cent of the men reported having a sexual problem.

A setting in which one would expect sexual difficulties to present relatively often is the *gynaecology clinic*. In the United States, Levine and Yost (1976) interviewed 59 black, largely lower-social-class women in the age range 30-39 who attended a gynaecology clinic for non-sexual complaints. Seventeen per cent were unable to achieve orgasm with a partner by any means. Most of these women had a history of adequate previous sexual function. In addition, a further one in five women who were able to achieve orgasm were not satisfied with their sexual relationships. The risk of sexual dysfunction was five times greater in women who had undergone pelvic surgery.

The prevalence of sexual dysfunction has also been investigated in patients attending a *clinic for sexually transmitted diseases* (Catalan *et al.* 1981). Semi-structured interviews with 70 male and 70 female clinic attenders revealed that almost a quarter of the men and two-fifths of the women were experiencing sexual dysfunction. The most frequent problems among the men were premature ejaculation (13 per cent), erectile dysfunction (7 per cent) and loss of libido (6 per cent). All but one man regarded the dysfunctions as a problem and would have liked help with them. The most common forms of sexual dysfunction among the women were 'coital orgasmic dysfunction' (37 per cent) and 'loss of libido' (13 per cent). All but two of the women with dysfunctions would have liked help for their sexual difficulties.

Swan and Wilson (1979) investigated 79 attenders at a *psychiatric clinic* who were married and living with their spouses, and had no previous history of psychiatric treatment. There were 63 women and 16 men. After an elaborate screening procedure, 12 per cent of the sample were identified as having sexual or marital problems for which it was considered that help could be, and was, offered. Unfortunately, the authors did not provide separate figures for sexual and marital problems.

The frequency of presentation of sexual difficulties in other clinical settings, such as the diabetic clinic, will be considered in Chapter 5.

Because of absence of control groups, these studies of sexual dysfunction among patients attending clinics of various kinds have not provided evidence that sexual problems occur more often in these patients than in the general population, although this may be the case. However, it should remind people who work in such clinics that patients may have sexual difficulties in addition to their presenting problems, and that the clinical interview provides an ideal opportunity to identify those who might wish for help. The patterns of sexual dysfunction in women and men attending medical clinics appear to mirror those found in general population surveys.

THE EFFECTS OF SEXUAL PROBLEMS

When looking for evidence concerning the effects of sexual problems on people's lives one is confronted by a paucity of information. In part this is because of the difficulty of distinguishing cause from effect. Thus it is often unclear whether non-sexual problems experienced by an individual or couple are the reasons for a sexual dysfunction, or whether they are the consequences of the sexual difficulty. We will focus on two areas, namely the effects of sexual problems on relationships in general, and the distress which is caused by such problems.

The effects on relationships

It was noted earlier that sexual difficulties need not necessarily cause general marital disharmony and dissatisfaction (Frank *et al.* 1978). Nevertheless, it is clear that very often couples with sexual problems do have unhappy marriages and that in this respect many couples who seek sex therapy resemble couples who seek marital therapy (Frank *et al.* 1976). Although, as discussed in the next chapter, sexual dysfunction will often be the direct consequence of general relationship problems, clinical experience also indicates that sexual disharmony is often the cause of unhappiness in a couple's general relationship. For example, in a marriage in which a man's erectile dysfunction or premature ejaculation has resulted in repeated frustration for both himself and his partner, this dissatisfaction is likely gradually to taint the rest of the relationship. Furthermore, many couples with sexual dysfunction cease talking about sexual matters and, in particular, about their wishes and expectations (p. 70). This impaired communication may gradually become a feature of the general relationship, leading to further resentment and loss of affection (although, as Hartman (1980) has shown, this is not necessarily the pattern in all couples with sexual difficulties). In a proportion of cases, the final outcome will be marital breakdown and divorce, sometimes preceded by violence as a result of jealousy. In a retrospective study, Thornes and Collard (1979) demonstrated that sexual dissatisfaction at the start of a marriage is associated with increased risk of the marriage ending in divorce. Alternatively, the relationship may continue, but be an extremely unhappy one for both partners. The immediate consequences of marital disharmony for children can be very serious (Stuart 1980). In addition, there are the possible longer-term consequences for a child whose primary model of how marital partners relate is characterized by lack of both affection and physical contact (p. 59).

The effects on the individual

Sexual dysfunction in individuals without partners may prevent them forming a relationship because of feelings of inadequacy, or fear of a partner's response to discovery of the problem. This situation is commonly seen in clinical practice. Fortunately, recent advances in treatment methods now enable one to offer help to individuals without partners (Chapter 14).

Emotional effects of sexual problems

Although the results from different studies are not totally consistent, there is substantial evidence suggesting that many individuals with sexual dysfunction are likely to experience reduced self-esteem, distress and, specifically, symptoms of depression and anxiety. Thus, although Maurice and Guze (1970) reported that few of their series of patient with sexual disorders also had psychiatric conditions (although many had a history of psychiatric illness), several other workers have produced evidence that a relatively high proportion of such patients experience psychiatric symptoms and suffer from psychiatric disorders (Derogatis *et al.* 1981; Meyer *et al.* 1975; O'Connor and Stern 1972). Once again we are faced with the difficulty of distinguishing cause from effect. Undoubtedly, in some patients where sexual and psychiatric disorders co-exist, the sexual problems are the result of the psychopathology (p. 73). Nevertheless, in many other cases, depression and anxiety will occur as a reaction to sexual dysfunction, and resolution of the latter will lead to relief of the symptoms.

CONCLUSIONS

In this chapter we have reviewed some of the available information concerning two questions relevant to the application of sex therapy, namely, how common are sexual problems? and what effects do they have? It is clear that sexual difficulties are experienced by many people in the general population, and that they tend to be reported more often by women than by men. The most common problem reported by women is impaired interest in sex. At least one in ten women never experience orgasm. Premature ejaculation is the problem most often reported by men. Erectile dysfunction occurs in less than 10 per cent of men, but the proportion increases with age. Very often sexual dysfunction does not cause sexual dissatisfaction, especially in men, nor does everyone with a sexual problem wish for help. However, the substantial proportion of people with problems who also want help is reflected in the large numbers of referrals to sexual dysfunction clinics.

We have also considered the prevalence of sexual problems in clinical settings, including general practice, clinics for urology, gynaecology, family planning, sexually transmitted diseases, and psychiatry. It is clear that patients with sexual difficulties are common in these settings. It should be relatively easy to identify such patients' sexual problems and arrange appropriate help if required.

Because of the difficulty encountered in trying to disentangle cause from effect, it is not easy to demonstrate the effects that sexual disorders have on people's lives. Some couples' relationships remain happy despite their sexual problems; however, sexual difficulties increase the risk of marital dissatisfaction and eventual divorce. Single people with sexual difficulties may avoid forming new relationships. Psychiatric symptoms are commonly associated with sexual problems. Sometimes this is because psychiatric disorder has caused the sexual problems, but often it is because the sexual difficulties themselves are causing distress.

5

Causes of sexual problems

In most cases more than one factor is relevant in causing a sexual problem. In addition, factors are often contributory rather than causal. Each by itself may not ensure the development of a sexual problem, but a problem may result from a complex interaction of factors. In couples this commonly reflects the characteristics both of each partner and of their relationship.

Broadly speaking the causes of sexual problems can be separated into those which are *psychological* and those which are *physical*. Physical causes may be sub-divided into *physical illness, surgery,* and *drugs* (prescribed and non-prescribed).

A useful way of further classifying causes of sexual dysfunction and their interactions is to differentiate them temporally. This can assist understanding of the mechanisms involved. Thus one can separate the causes into:

(1) *predisposing factors*, which include experiences early in life which have made a person vulnerable to developing sexual difficulties at a later stage;

(2) *precipitants*, which are events or experiences associated with the initial appearance of a dysfunction; and

(3) *maintaining factors*, which explain why a dysfunction persists.

Many of the factors which will be discussed within this chapter are based on surmise and clinical impression. It is difficult to demonstrate conclusively that some of the possible causes are relevant, especially those which may have occurred many years earlier in an individual's development. Even with organic factors there are numerous examples of controversy concerning whether, and how, such factors contribute to sexual dysfunction. Furthermore, the causes of a sexual problem may remain obscure even after a thorough assessment, though in many cases the individual or couple may still be offered treatment. The therapist should discuss with the clients hypotheses concerning the likely causes of the problem, explaining that it should be possible to verify or refute the formulation as treatment proceeds.

PSYCHOLOGICAL CAUSES

The range of psychological factors relevant to the aetiology of sexual dysfunction is enormous, and differentiation of them is to some extent arbitrary. Considering causes of sexual dysfunction in terms of predisposing factors, precipitants, and maintaining factors is particularly pertinent when reviewing psychological causes. The causes that will be considered here are summarized in Table 5.1.

TABLE 5.1

Psychological causes of sexual dysfunction

Predisposing factors	
	Traumatic early sexual experiences
Restrictive upbringing	Early insecurity in psychosexual role
Disturbed family relationships	
Inadequate sexual information	
Precipitants	
	Reaction to organic factors
Childbirth	Ageing
Discord in the general relationship	Depression and anxiety
Infidelity	Traumatic sexual experience
Unreasonable expectations	
Dysfunction in the partner	
Random failure	
Maintaining factors	
	Fear of intimacy
Performance anxiety	Impaired self-image
Anticipation of failure	Inadequate sexual information;
Guilt	sexual myths
Loss of attraction between partners	Restricted foreplay
Poor communication between	Psychiatric disorder
partners	
Discord in the general relationship	

Predisposing factors

These are the factors whose recognition is most likely to be conjectural, because early experiences tend to be easily forgotten or
distorted in the light of subsequent events. However, it is important to try to identify predisposing factors as their recognition
can help the patient (and the therapist) make sense of the current
difficulties. Sometimes, particularly in the case of primary disorders (p. 31), identification of early experiences will be the
most important step in understanding the sexual problem. Subsequent management will depend on altering the factors which
now maintain the dysfunction, including current attitudes
towards sexuality.

Restrictive upbringing.   A child's experience of his or her family's
attitudes towards sexuality and personal relationships is likely to
have a profound effect on later psychosexual development. Such
attitudes may be expressed covertly or overtly. Thus, in many
families, sex is never discussed and, because it is a taboo subject,
becomes regarded by a child as something which must in some
way be wrong or shameful. In other families, parents may openly
express their negative attitudes towards sexuality. For example,
a girl's mother may encourage her daughter to regard sex as a
chore which must be undertaken in order to please her partner
and to obtain the benefits of a marital relationship. The girl may
be given the impression by her mother that sexual intercourse
involves pain. A boy may be encouraged to regard women who
enjoy sex as disreputable, so that he may develop a double-
standard towards women—the notion of the 'good' woman who
is not sexual, or at least keeps her sexuality under a tight rein,
and who will make a suitable marital partner, and the 'bad' woman
who actively enjoys and seeks out sexual experience, but who
should be avoided at all costs when it comes to finding a permanent
mate.

   It takes little imagination to see how exposure to such negative
attitudes can contribute to the later development of sexual dysfunction. If a woman has been brought up to regard sex as a
necessary chore she may feel guilty about her desires for, or
enjoyment of, sexual relationships, and this may therefore inhibit
her sexual responsiveness. The expectation that sexual inter-

course will be a painful experience might contribute to the development of vaginismus. A double-standard towards female sexuality may lead a boy to seek out a non-responsive partner, or he may experience revulsion when he discovers that his partner's level of sexual desire is equivalent to his own. He is also likely to treat disparagingly partners who are sexually responsive.

Disturbed family relationships. How children perceive their parents' relationships, and the relationships children have with their parents, are also likely to be important in determining vulnerability to later sexual and other interpersonal difficulties. If the relationship between parents is characterized by friction and lack of affection, especially physical affection, a child is presented with a poor initial model for men/women relationships. Similarly, if the relationship between the child and either parent is lacking in warmth and affection, difficulties in establishing intimate relationships in adulthood may be created. One would predict that the relationship with the opposite-sex parent would be most important in this respect.

The theoretical implications of disturbed family relationships are supported by clinical impression, but unfortunately there is only scanty research evidence. In a series of patients assessed for treatment of sexual dysfunction, O'Connor and Stern (1972) found that a history of death of either a parent or a sibling was more common than expected, and also that 23 per cent of patients had experienced separation of their parents. In a study of married Swedish women by Uddenberg (1974), subjects who were infrequently or never orgasmic generally reported less satisfactory relationships with their fathers during childhood than women with good orgasmic frequency. Similarly, women who were dissatisfied with their sexual relationships reported poorer relationships with their fathers during adolescence than those satisfied with their sexual relationships. Fisher (1973) found that women with 'good orgasmic consistency' less often recalled loss or separation of their parents than those women with unsatisfactory orgasmic function. Finally, in their study of Swedish married men (p. 48), Nettelbladt and Uddenberg (1979) found that, when compared with men with good sexual adjustment, those with sexual dysfunction more often described their fathers negatively, and reported contact with them during childhood and adolescence as being poor and relatively infrequent. They also more often reported infrequent and poor contact with their mothers during adolescence (but not during childhood), and tended to characterize their mothers as dominating.

Thus, there appears to be some tentative evidence for the theories and clinical impressions discussed earlier. However, one must interpret very cautiously evidence based on retrospective inquiries, because of the possible distortion of memory in the light of subsequent experiences. In addition, they tell us little about causal mechanisms. For example, rather than having a direct effect on sexuality, poor parent-child relationships might cause sexual difficulties through their effects on self-esteem or the ability to cope with intimacy.

Inadequate sexual information. Although there is a lack of empirical evidence, clinical impression suggests that inadequate or poor information about sexuality is an important vulnerability factor for the development of sexual dysfunction. Sex education has been woefully inadequate or entirely lacking for many people, especially those now of middle or older age. In many cases sexual information will be based to a large extent on dirty jokes heard in adolescence, or on poor information gained from discussion with other children whose sex education has been equally inadequate. Lack of knowledge about sexual anatomy may lead to sexual dysfunction. For example, if a woman does not know the position of the clitoris, or does not even know that it exists, she may be vulnerable to orgasmic dysfunction; similar ignorance on the part of a man may contribute to sexual dysfunction in his partner. Knowledge of sexuality is often particularly poor concerning the opposite sex.

Inadequate sex education can contribute to belief in some of the *sexual myths*, of which examples are given in Table 5.2. At least one of these myths (no. 10) has been promoted by a marriage manual which was very popular until quite recently (Van de Velde 1930). The expectations created by such a belief can impose great demands on a sexual relationship.

Traumatic early sexual experiences. It is unclear to what extent unpleasant childhood sexual experiences contribute to the development of sexual difficulties in later life. Childhood sexual experi-

TABLE 5.2

Some common sexual myths

1. A man always wants and is always ready to have sex
2. Sex must only ever occur at the instigation of the man
3. Any woman who initiates sex is immoral
4. Sex equals intercourse: anything else doesn't really count
5. When a man gets an erection it is bad for him not to use it to get an orgasm very soon
6. Sex should always be natural and spontaneous: thinking or talking about it spoils it
7. All physical contact must lead to intercourse
8. Men should not express their feelings
9. Any man ought to know how to give pleasure to any woman
10. Sex is really good only when partners have orgasms simultaneously
11. If people love each other they will know how to enjoy sex together
12. Partners in a sexual relationship instinctively know what the other partner thinks or wants
13. Masturbation is dirty or harmful
14. Masturbation within a sexual relationship is wrong
15. If a man loses his erection it means he doesn't find his partner attractive
16. It is wrong to have fantasies during intercourse
17. A man cannot say 'no' to sex/a woman cannot say 'no' to sex
18. There are certain absolute, universal rules about what is normal in sex.

ences, especially incest, are far more common than previously recognized. Following their study of male sexuality, Kinsey and colleagues (1948) reported that incestuous experiences with older persons were rare; among women they found that 4 per cent reported pre-adolescent sexual approaches by their fathers (Kinsey *et al.* 1953). More recently, of 952 college students in the USA asked about pre-pubertal sexual activity with adults, 7.7 per cent of the women and 4.8 per cent of the men reported such an experience (Fritz *et al.* 1981). The girls' experiences in nine out of ten cases were of a heterosexual nature, whereas 40 per cent of the experiences of the males were homosexual. When Finkelhor (1980) asked 796 New England college students about sexual experiences with siblings, 15 per cent of the women and 10 per cent of the men reported some type of sexual experience involving a brother or sister. Usually the experiences were of an exploratory nature (e.g. general fondling, and touching of the genitals).

Little information is available concerning how often such experiences are associated with subsequent sexual problems, and there is only scanty information concerning the type of sexual experience most likely to have such an association (Mrazek and Mrazek 1981). In the study by Fritz *et al.* (1981), 23 per cent of the women who had been 'sexually molested' in childhood by adults reported problems in their current sexual adjustment, whereas only 10 per cent of the boys who had experienced such activities reported difficulties. Unfortunately, no information was provided concerning sexual problems among those who had *not* been molested. The authors commented that the girls more often regarded the sexual experiences as having been a personal violation, whereas the reactions of the boys were more often neutral, or even positive, as if the act was viewed in many cases as an initiation. Those women who thought they had succumbed to the sexual experience as a result of persuasion (i.e. without force or threat being used) were more likely to report current sexual difficulties.

Finkelhor (1980) did not report how many of the subjects in his study now had sexual difficulties. However, among the women he found that when the early sexual experience had been with an older sibling, or it had been forced on the individual (a quarter of cases), current sexual self-esteem was in general lower than among other female students who had not experienced sibling sex. Interestingly, when the sibling sexual activity had occurred after the age of nine and was recalled as a positive experience, current sexual self-esteem was higher than among women who had not experienced sibling sexual activity. Finkelhor did not consider the possibility that the memories of the early sexual experiences might have been modified in the light of current sexual adjustment. He concluded that sexual activity with a sibling does not usually have devastating effects on subsequent sexual adjustment unless exploitation and force have been used.

Finally, Tsai *et al.* (1979) compared three groups of women with regard to 'sexual molestation' in childhood: first, a clinical group of women who had sought help with problems associated with childhood sexual molestation; secondly, a non-clinical group of women who as children had been molested but who considered themselves to be well-adjusted; and, thirdly, a control group of women who had never been molested. As expected, the clinical group differed from both the other two groups on several measures of general and sexual adjustment, there being little difference between the non-clinical and control groups. The most interesting findings concerned the differences in the molestation experiences of the clinical and the non-clinical groups. Thus in the clinical group: (1) more had been molested at an older age, especially after the age of 11; (2) stronger emotional experiences at the time of the molestation were reported, including greater pressure to participate, greater pain, and greater dislike for the molester; and (3) sexual molestation occurred more frequently and over a longer period.

In summary, it seems that childhood sexual experiences, especially in women, can be associated with subsequent sexual difficulties, but it is unclear how often this happens. A study of college women suggests that difficulties occur in a minority of cases. The research findings at present suggest that later sexual difficulties are more likely if the experience involved threats or force, occurred at an older age (when greater awareness of the implication of the behaviour may cause more guilt), was associated with strong negative emotional feelings, and took place persistently. A further important feature will undoubtedly be the quality of subsequent sexual encounters; positive experiences are likely to negate the effects of early sexual traumas, whereas adverse experiences are likely to reinforce such effects.

Early insecurity in psychosexual role. Lack of security or comfort with personal sexuality may predispose to sexual dysfunction. The term 'personal sexuality' refers to the attitudes of people towards their own bodies, especially their sexual anatomy, and towards their sexual thoughts and urges. Many factors will influence the development of ease or discomfort with personal sexuality but early experiences are especially important. Timing of puberty is one example. If a young person develops physical characteristics earlier than others of the same age, embarrassment may persist into adolescence. For example, a girl whose breast development pre-dates that of most other girls of the same age may be teased and become self-conscious about her breasts. Similarly, delayed puberty can cause feelings of inadequacy. Family attitudes to the adolescent's emerging sexuality are also likely to influence psychosexual adjustment. If parents encourage the adolescent to persist with pre-pubertal activities and fail to acknowledge the adolescent's new needs, including those of privacy, this may cause the young person to feel that sexual development is unwelcome, and that it should be denied or suppressed. The consequent uneasiness with sexuality may persist into adulthood. Furthermore, religious beliefs may compound the adolescent's confusion about sexuality, particularly when strong sexual urges, which appear to conflict with religious ideals, are experienced.

Precipitants

Sexual dysfunction often seems to be precipitated by a particular experience. A woman with vaginismus whose problem began after she was shocked by the size of the first erection she witnessed provides an obvious sample. Generally, precipitants are less commonly identified for primary dysfunctions. For example, premature ejaculation may gradually develop into a problem, without a clear precipitant, when a man fails to gain ejaculatory control after experiencing, as do many young men, rapid ejaculation during his first sexual experiences.

Some of the more common psychological precipitants of sexual dysfunction are considered below (see Table 5.1). Physical disorders, medication and drugs, which are also important precipitants, are considered later in this chapter.

Childbirth.   Secondary loss of interest in sex in women often follows childbirth. Only rarely does this appear to result from the stress of childbirth itself. More often a woman's interest in sex fails to return after childbirth because of depression, tiredness, and the stresses of coping with a young baby. In addition, soreness of an episiotomy scar, or post-partum vaginal dryness (particularly in breast-feeding mothers), may make sexual intercourse uncomfortable and therefore lead to avoidance or reduced interest. A clinical impression is that sexual difficulties most commonly follow the birth of a second baby. Why this should be so is unclear. Many couples find that the arrival of a second child poses considerable extra demands, and often causes chronic tiredness. Furthermore, if a couple have decided to limit their family to two children and either partner has difficulty in accepting sexuality when there is no chance of conception, this could also be a contributory factor.

Discord in the general relationship. As has already been noted, and will be emphasized again elsewhere in this book, discord in a couple's relationship is the most common reason for sexual dysfunction, both as a precipitant and a maintaining factor. Although some couples are able to continue a satisfactory sexual relationship in spite of considerable general friction, this is unusual. The next chapter will emphasize the necessity to identify during the assessment couples whose sexual problems are symptomatic of difficulties in their relationship in general. Unfortunately, this is not always easy. Whereas chronic hostility and dislike may be very apparent, loss of affection, or unexpressed resentment may be denied by a couple.

Infidelity. Discovery of a partner's infidelity is a fairly common precipitant of sexual dysfunction, especially loss of interest in sex or erectile dysfunction. Guilt concerning secret infidelity may also precipitate dysfunction in the unfaithful partner. Infidelity will in itself often reflect other problems in the relationship. Sometimes, a person first recognizes sexual dysfunction following a more satisfactory sexual experience with a new partner.

Unreasonable expectations. An individual's sexual expectations will partly determine current satisfaction. Unreasonable expectations may cause problems and precipitate apparent dysfunction. One recent example was the publicity concerning multiple orgasms in women. This has caused some women to think that they were inadequate because they experienced orgasm only once during sexual activity. Another example was the controversy over the apparent difference, particularly in terms of sexual maturity, between 'clitoral' and 'vaginal' orgasms. As noted in Chapter 2, this sexual myth was firmly refuted by Master and Johnson's studies of female sexual response.

Dysfunction in the partner. Sexual dysfunction may be precipitated by dysfunction in the partner. For example, female orgasmic dysfunction or impaired sexual interest are often associated with premature ejaculation or erectile dysfunction. The nature of the association can be in either direction. Thus a man whose partner loses interest in sex may develop premature ejaculation, and a woman whose partner develops erectile dysfunction may lose interest in sex. In such cases it is important to determine which dysfunction developed first because this usually should be the initial focus of treatment. Among couples accepted for sex therapy, sexual dysfunction is found in both partners in a third or more cases (p. 42).

Random failure. An isolated experience of failure can sometimes precipitate sexual dysfunction because of the psychological sequelae of such an episode. For example, a middle-aged man whose alcohol consumption has recently increased markedly in response to stress at work might find after an evening's particularly heavy drinking that he cannot make love to his wife because of failure to get an erection. Subsequently, perhaps again under the influence of alcohol, he may be tense and strive to get an erection because of his fear of further failure. Another failure can set up a vicious circle of fear of failure, performance anxiety, and actual failure, thus leading to persistent erectile dysfunction.

Reaction to organic factors. Psychological responses to major illness or surgery can be extremely important in determining subsequent sexual adjustment. As this is discussed later in this chapter (p. 77), two brief examples will suffice. After a heart attack a man (or woman) may develop sexual dysfunction because, in the absence of medical advice (Krop *et al.* 1979), he fears that a further attack is likely to be precipitated by sexual intercourse (Mehta and Krop 1979). Following mastectomy for breast cancer as many as one-third of women have serious sexual difficulties one year later (Maguire *et al.* 1978). Difficulties are likely to result from a sense of loss of sexual attractiveness, depression, or revulsion experienced by the woman's partner.

Ageing. The sexual effects of ageing were discussed in Chapter 2. An individual's reactions to these changes will be the main determinants of whether sexual dysfunction develops. For example, a woman may lose her interest in sex because she feels embarrassed when, following the menopause, she experiences only slight lubrication during foreplay. Similarly, if a middle-aged man becomes concerned because he requires more stimulation than he used to in order to keep his erection and to ejaculate, erectile dysfunction may result.

Several other factors can contribute to the association between ageing and the development of sexual dysfunction. First, general physical changes may contribute to loss of attractiveness, or to an individual's sense of unattractiveness. These include, for example, weight gain, impaired mobility, and sagging breasts. Secondly, those physical illnesses which are likely to impair sexual function become more common in older age. These include cardiovascular disease, degenerative disorders of the joints, parkinsonism, and malignant disease. Thirdly, and as a result of the increased incidence of disease, the use of medication likely to affect sexual function (p. 79) increases with age. Fourthly, psychiatric disorders, especially depression, anxiety, and dementia become more common, and all three, together with the drugs used to treat them, are likely to affect sexual interest and function. Furthermore, some 'sexual myths' which reflect attitudes to sexuality in older people may contribute to the development of sexual dysfunction. These include the following: (1) sex is the prerogative of the young and attractive; (2) sex should cease when procreation is no longer possible; and (3) sexual performance usually ceases after middle age, and, if it does not, this is abnormal.

Depression and anxiety. The role of psychiatric disorders in causing sexual dysfunction will be discussed later (p. 73). Depression is a particularly important precipitant for sexual dysfunction, especially impaired interest in sex.

Traumatic sexual experience. Surprisingly little information is available to support the widely accepted notion that sexual trauma often precipitates sexual dysfunction. The most obvious example is rape. There is some evidence that many female rape victims gain less satisfaction from sex after the assault, have sexual intercourse less often, and are at risk of developing problems concerning sexual desire, sexual arousal, and orgasm (Burgess and Holmstrom 1979; Feldman-Summers *et al.* 1979; Becker *et al.* 1982). Phobic aversion to sexual activity has also been reported as being common among rape victims (Becker *et al.* 1982). Interestingly, Feldman-Summers *et al.* (1979) found that decreased sexual satisfaction after rape primarily affected sexual behaviours likely to have occurred during the assault, such as intercourse, touching of genitals, and visual exposure to male genitals, but behaviours not usually involved in rape, such as self-masturbation and showing and receiving affection, remained unaffected.

Unwanted pregnancy is another form of sexual trauma which may lead to subsequent avoidance of, or loss of desire for, sexual activity. However, it is not known how often sexual problems follow unwanted pregnancies.

Maintaining factors

The factors which sustain sexual problems are the most important when it comes to treatment (Table 5.1). Only maintaining factors are directly amenable to modification. Thus, although past events affect current attitudes and emotional responses, and during therapy a person may explore such experiences, any changes which occur will result from modification of current attitudes through re-evaluation of the past.

When considering some of the factors which may contribute to the maintenance of sexual difficulties it is worth noting that anxiety is a factor common to several of them. The explanation is very simple: anxiety and sexual interest and response are largely incompatible. Whatever the cause of anxiety, it can affect sexual function by leading to avoidance, lack of drive, inhibited arousal, or disturbance of orgasm. Some people clearly recognize their anxiety during sexual activity. Others may notice a sense of detachment from the sexual experience, almost as if they had become uninvolved observers. Masters and Johnson (1970) have called this experience 'spectatoring'. Feelings of boredom or irritation may also reflect anxiety.

Performance anxiety. Obsessive concern with adequate sexual performance is one of the most common reasons for the persistence of sexual dysfunction. This applies especially to men with erectile difficulties or premature ejaculation, and women with orgasmic dysfunction. For example, a man with erectile dysfunction may be concerned above all else with whether or not he can get an erection and, if he does, with keeping it long enough for sexual intercourse to occur and his partner to be satisfied. He may try to 'will' his erection, rather than allow it to occur as a natural response to erotic pleasure. He may also become very anxious at the point of vaginal penetration when he feels most need to maintain his erection. These anxieties ensure that he continues to experience erectile difficulties and, as often happens, that the problem worsens. A similar pattern may apply to a woman who has difficulty reaching orgasm. She may have thoughts such as 'my partner will get tired of stimulating me if I do not come soon', or 'he won't think much of me if I do not have an orgasm', or 'it will hurt his pride if I do not have a climax'. In view of such thoughts, and the excessive demand that some men place on their partners to achieve orgasm in order to satisfy their own performance needs, it is not surprising that many women resort to faking orgasms.

Performance anxiety is thus related to an excessive need to perform or to satisfy the partner, with little heed being paid to the individual's own pleasure and satisfaction. Sex therapy aims to encourage partners to be more selfish and to abandon themselves to their erotic sexual experience, rather than being constrained by performance needs.

Anticipation of failure. Closely related to performance anxiety is the anticipation that most couples with sexual dysfunction develop about the likely outcome of each sexual experience. Thus, as one failure follows another, a couple eventually expect failure. A vicious circle is established which either leads to persistence of the problem, or eventual cessation of sexual activity altogether.

Guilt. This is a common feeling experienced by people with sexual problems. It may reflect long-standing inhibitions about sex resulting, for example, from a restrictive upbringing (p. 58). Abandonment to erotic pleasure may therefore be impossible. Guilt may also be experienced because of the perceived effects of sexual dysfunction on the partner. For example, a woman who has lost interest in sex following childbirth may nevertheless have sexual intercourse because she feels guilty about denying her partner sexual satisfaction. However, this may make her resentful and therefore hinder normal recovery of her sexual interest.

Loss of attraction between partners. This is often reflected in sexual dysfunction. The change may have occurred spontaneously, or might reflect other emotional or social factors, ageing, or physical changes (e.g. obesity, poor hygiene, mutilating surgery).

Poor communication between partners. Many couples who develop sexual dysfunction are unable to discuss their sexual relationship. Consequently, not only are the partners unable to express their sexual needs and anxieties, but they may each begin to guess what the other is thinking and feeling. Such guessing can lead to serious misconceptions and further contribute to the sexual difficulties. For example, a woman whose interest in sex is reduced following childbirth may find it impossible to tell her partner that she now requires more gentle caressing before she can begin to get aroused. Her partner may mistake her reduced enthusiasm for sex as a personal rejection and start to withdraw from lovemaking, or, when lovemaking does occur, hurry the act because he believes his partner wants him to get it over quickly. Communication difficulties should be tackled early in sex therapy.

Discord in the general relationship. Just as disturbance in the general relationship between partners is a common precipitant of sexual dysfunction, so continuing disharmony is a very important maintaining factor. For most couples, sexuality, affection, trust, and general harmony are tightly intertwined, a disturbance in one of these factors affecting all the others. A satisfactory sexual relationship usually cannot be maintained if either partner is feeling very resentful towards, or has lost all affection for, the other partner. Bancroft (1983) reported that sexual dysfunction was certainly secondary to general relationship problems in 17 per cent of men and 24 per cent of women referred to a sexual dysfunction clinic in Edinburgh. Therapists often have difficulty in deciding how sound a couple's relationship is in general; in 47 per cent of the cases in which the man presented to the clinic in Edinburgh and in 32 per cent of those in which the woman presented it was 'uncertain' whether the sexual dysfunction was secondary to relationship problems. Serious general relationship problems preclude sex therapy, but less serious problems can often be dealt with during sex therapy provided the problems are not overwhelming and there are sufficient positive feelings between the partners (Chapter 11).

Fear of intimacy. Fear of intimacy is a common cause of sexual problems (Kaplan 1977; 1979). Intimacy has been defined as 'a special quality of emotional closeness between two people . . . an affectionate bond . . . composed of mutual caring, responsibility, trust, open-communication of feelings and sensations, as well as the non-defended interchange of information about significant emotional events' (Kaplan 1979). In relationships where there is a high degree of intimacy there is also likely to be sexual happiness because the partners are able to be open with each other, and to abandon themselves to erotic pleasure. We have already noted that individuals who find difficulty in coping with intimacy often come from backgrounds characterized by a lack of warmth and affection. Kaplan believes that a single person who has intimacy problems is likely to have a succession of relationships, each of which ends at the same point of closeness when the individual destroys the relationship because further involvement is too threatening. In couples this problem usually results in one or both partners failing to engage wholeheartedly in the sexual relationship. One partner may always rush any sexual act to a conclusion because the closeness of mutual caressing and arousal is threatening. Fear of intimacy is thus an important factor in the maintenance of sexual dysfunction; if unresolved it is likely to lead to both persistent and worsening difficulties. If fear of intimacy is contributing to a couple's sexual problems this will usually become obvious during the early stages of sex therapy when the couple are asked to begin the pleasuring exercises (p. 128).

Impaired self-image. Once a sexual dysfunction is established, the secondary effect of this on an individual's self-image may maintain the problem or make it worse. For example, a man's sense of masculinity may be undermined by erectile dysfunction. Anxiety provoked by such feelings may compound the erectile difficulty. Similarly, a woman who never reaches orgasm during sex with a partner may feel that she is not a complete woman. It is not always the individual with the dysfunction who experiences poor self-image. Thus a woman who fakes orgasm may be realistically aware of how important it is to her partner's self-esteem that she should achieve orgasm. Similarly, the partner of a man with erectile dysfunction may feel the problem is the result of him finding her unattractive.

Dissatisfaction with body image may contribute to the persistence of sexual dysfunction. For example, a woman who feels that her breasts or abdomen are much too large may find it impossible to abandon herself to her partner's caresses. In therapy, people are sometimes helped to develop a more rational appraisal of their bodies (p. 217). Quite often, very specific disturbance of body image contribute to a dysfunction. For example, a woman with vaginismus may have distorted ideas about her genitals, particularly in terms of their appearance, size, and cleanliness.

Inadequate sexual information; sexual myths.   Just as inadequate as misguided information about sexuality makes a person vulnerable to sexual dysfunction, so these factors can also contribute to the persistence of a problem once it develops. When communication between partners is also poor, an important means of correcting misinformation or making new discoveries about the partner is lost. Lack of confidence may further compound the problem. For example, a woman who fails to get fully aroused or be orgasmic with her partner because he, out of ignorance, never provides her with clitoral stimulation, may feel unable to tell her partner of her needs, partly because they no longer (or never did) discuss their sexual relationship and partly because she fears she may hurt his pride by suggesting he is anything less than a perfect lover. Belief in some of the sexual myths which were discussed earlier (Table 5.2) may also serve to perpetuate a dysfunction.

Restricted foreplay.   A sexual problem may first develop and then persist because a couple engage in little or no foreplay before sexual intercourse. Also, couples with sexual difficulties often spend less and less time on foreplay before sexual intercourse. This may occur for several reasons. A woman who has lost most or all of her interest in sex may feel she must have sex for her partner's sake, but finish it as quickly as possible. It is increasingly unlikely, therefore, that she will get pleasure from the sexual relationship and so her interest usually declines even further. A man with premature ejaculation may avoid foreplay because he fears this will lead to his becoming too aroused and therefore ejaculating more quickly. This usually results in little or no pleasure for both the man and his partner, thus adding further tension to the sexual relationship and making the problem worse. The sensate focus exercises used in sex therapy are intended to encourage full, relaxed, and enjoyable foreplay.

Psychiatric disorder. Many people suffering from *depression* experience loss of interest in sex (Beck 1967). Fewer experience impaired sexual performance (Mathew and Weinmann 1982). Thus Weissman and Paykel (1974) found that the most marked difference between depressed and non-depressed women in terms of their sexuality was the extent to which the depressed women reported impaired sexual interest. Their actual frequency of sexual intercourse was less markedly affected by the mood disturbance. A few women reported orgasmic dysfunction or dyspareunia. On recovery from depression the only major change in sexual adjustment was increased interest in sex. Beaumont (1977) also found that 'impaired libido' was the most common effect of depression in men and women, with one-fifth of subjects having ceased sexual intercourse altogether after becoming depressed. A few depressed men suffered erectile dysfunction and some women reported difficulty in reaching orgasm.

Account must be taken of the possible deleterious side-effects of antidepressants (Table 5.5). For example, in the study of Beaumont (1977) mentioned above, once antidepressant therapy (with clomipramine) was started, further changes in sexual function occurred and these usually affected sexual performance. One-fifth of the men developed erectile difficulties and a few more women now reported failure to experience orgasm. Some women, however, reported improvement in their sexual responsiveness when taking the antidepressant, presumably because of the beneficial effects of the medication on their mood.

In *mania* and *hypomania* there is often a marked increase in sexual interest, sometimes causing disinhibition and promiscuity. However, sexual interest is occasionally impaired (Winokur *et al.* 1969). Lithium carbonate, which is often used to reduce the likelihood of further manic-depressive episodes, appears to reduce sexual interest in some people (Vinarova *et al* 1972). Whether this is because of the damping down of mood fluctuations or a direct physiological effect is not known.

Diminution of interest in sex often accompanies *schizophrenia*, especially in patients with severe chronic psychopathology (Lyketsos *et al.* 1983). Phenothiazines (especially thioridazine), which are commonly used to treat this condition, can also have disruptive sexual side-effects (Table 5.5).

Little is known about how *anxiety states* affect sexuality. A surprising impression from the literature is that any effects are not very profound, certainly when compared with those of depression. This may be because it is anxiety about sexuality, rather than general anxiety, which is important in causing sexual problems.

In women suffering from *anorexia nervosa*, lack of interest in sex and orgasmic dysfunction are thought to be common (Kolodny *et al.* 1979). The disorder is often said to result from a dislike of the mature adult female body form, and is associated with marked disturbances of sex hormones (Crisp 1967). However, the deleterious effects of anorexia nervosa on sexuality may not affect all sufferers (Beaumont *et al.* 1981). Anorexia nervosa in men, a rare condition, is associated with considerable disturbance of sex hormone levels and therefore of sexual interest (Beaumont *et al.* 1972; McNab and Hawton 1981).

Alcoholism can have devastating effects on sexuality, for both psychological and physical reasons. Although Lemere and Smith (1973) estimated that only 8 per cent of male alcoholics of all ages seen by them had developed erectile dysfunction, Jensen (1979) found sexual dysfunction in 63 per cent of young male alcoholics. The most common dysfunction was reduced interest in sex (36 per cent). Erectile dysfunction (28 per cent), retarded ejaculation (16 per cent), and premature ejaculation (10 per cent) were also common. Among chronic alcoholics, Van Thiel and Lester (1976) found decreased sex drive and erectile dysfunction in as many as 80 per cent of cases. The reasons for such widespread sexual difficulties among alcoholics are probably three-fold. First, there are the serious effects the disorder can have on psychosocial adjustment, particularly on the relationship between the alcoholic and his or her partner. These include, for example, dislike of sexual activity with a habitually drunken partner, and morbid jealousy. Secondly, peripheral neuropathy, including involvement of the nerves concerned with sexual response, is a common complication of chronic alcoholism. Thirdly, disturbances in sex hormones are often found in alcoholics (Van Thiel and Lester 1976; 1979). These include abnormalities in oestrogen metabolism, inhibition

of gonadotrophin and testosterone production, and hyperprolactinaemia.
Some of the sexual problems associated with *drug addiction* are considered later (p. 83).

PHYSICAL CAUSES

Sex therapy was developed partly because it appeared that the majority of cases of sexual dysfunction were caused by psychological factors. This is certainly true for most types of sexual dysfunction, particularly premature ejaculation and orgasmic dysfunction. However, in recent years there has been increasing recognition of the role that a range of physical factors can play, especially in erectile disorders. In a study by Spark *et al.* (1980), for example, more than a third of 105 men with erectile dysfunction screened for endocrine disorder were found to have hormonal abnormalities. Although it is unclear how this series of men was identified, and the proportion of cases in which there was an hormonal abnormality is considerably in excess of that found in men usually referred to sexual dysfunction clinics, this study emphasizes the need to be alert for hormonal disturbance in this condition. In addition to neurological causes which have been known for a long while, further organic causes of erectile dysfunction, especially those involving the blood supply to and within the penis (Wagner and Green 1981; Michal 1982), are now being recognized.

Sexual dysfunction is also associated with many forms of physical illness, surgery, and medication. Clearly, anyone suffering from malaise resulting from illness or its treatment is unlikely to have much interest in sex. Broadly speaking there are five types of more specific association:
1. The physical condition or treatment may *directly interfere with physiological or anatomical mechanisms* involved in sexual interest, arousal or orgasm (e.g. pituitary tumours, diabetes, rectal surgery). Included here are disorders of the muscles or joints which affect mobility, or cause pain, and thereby impair sexual function.
2. Sexual dysfunction may occur because of a *psychological reaction to a physical condition or treatment* (e.g. myocardial infarction, mastectomy).

3. Sexual dysfunction may result from a *combination of physical and psychological factors*. This picture is common. For example, an adverse reaction to mild impairment of erectile capacity because of early diabetic peripheral neuropathy or multiple sclerosis may precipitate more severe or total erectile dysfunction.

4. *Illness or surgery may bring to light pre-existing sexual problems.* It should not be assumed that the co-existence of physical problems and sexual dysfunction always indicates a causal connection. This was illustrated by studies in which it was found that both men and women who suffered heart attacks had more often experienced sexual difficulties *before* the attacks than had control groups of people who had not had heart attacks (Abramov 1976; Wabrek and Burchell 1980).

5. *Sexual dysfunction caused by psychological factors may present under the guise of physical complaints*, especially in the gynaecology or family planning clinic, or in general practice. Doctors should be alert to such a possibility when faced, for example, by a woman who complains of vaginal discharge when no abnormality can be detected, or one who expresses dissatisfaction with whatever type of oral contraception is prescribed.

The rest of this chapter is devoted to the effects that physical illness and surgery can have on sexuality, and to the sexual side-effects of prescribed and non-prescribed drugs. The aetiological scheme used when considering psychological causes (i.e. distinguishing predisposing, precipitating, and maintaining factors) should also be used when assessing people with sexual problems resulting from physical disorders or treatments. However, as most physical factors can act in different people as predisposing factors, precipitants, or maintaining factors, this scheme is not used in the following sections.

PHYSICAL ILLNESS AND SURGERY

Some of the known effects on sexuality of physical illnesses and surgery are summarized at the end of this chapter in Tables 5.3 and 5.4 respectively. Therapists should be aware of such associations because people with undetected physical disorders may seek sex therapy. It is also important to understand how recognized illnesses can interfere with sexual function. Sex therapy and brief counselling are often of value for sexual problems caused by physical illness. This is often discussed in Chapter 14.

Unfortunately, it is often unclear in an individual case to what extent sexual dysfunction is the result of physical pathology and how much it is the result of psychological reactions to the physical disorder. Diabetes provides a good example. At one time it was thought that the distinction between erectile dysfunction of organic origin and that resulting from psychological factors was relatively straightforward. Recent investigation of diabetic men with erectile difficulties has cast doubt on this notion. For example, Fairburn *et al.* (1982) found an extremely varied clinical picture of erectile dysfunction in a series of 27 diabetic men. Over half the men experienced morning erections, and a third had spontaneous erections, both features generally being regarded as characteristic of psychological erectile dysfunction.

It is important to be aware of the possible psychological reactions to serious physical illness and chronic disability. The main factors to consider are: the reactions of the afflicted individual, the reactions of the partner, the nature of their relationship, and the response of the medical profession.

The reactions of the individual

1. *Anticipation of failure.* A person may believe that illness or surgery has destroyed his or her sexual capacity. This may be reinforced by the cultural stereotype of the 'sexless invalid' in which sex is viewed primarily as an activity for the youthful and attractive members of society. Although physical effects of surgery or illness on sexual function are often only transient, they may become permanent if an individual anticipates failure, or if a specific aspect of sexual function remains impaired. Lack of confidence may prevent resumption of sexual activity. A problem such as retrograde ejaculation following prostatectomy or phenothiazine usage may cause concern about overall sexual performance and thereby lead to avoidance of sex.

2. *Anticipation of harm or pain.* Fear of the consequences of sexual activity can also lead to avoidance. A person who has had a heart attack may fear relapse, or even sudden death (Bloch *et al.* 1975). Patients who have undergone renal transplantation or prostatectomy sometimes fear that damage will occur during

sexual activity. Similarly, anticipation of pain in patients with arthritic conditions may cause avoidance of sex.

3. *Impairment of self-concept.* An individual's sense of sexual attractiveness to others can be affected by illness or surgery. This is particularly likely if sexual anatomy has been altered (e.g. mastectomy, hysterectomy), or if other parts of the body have been changed (e.g. amputation, severe burns, or loss of mobility).

4. *Depression.* Illness or surgery may precipitate depression. This can be the result of chronic pain, forced change in lifestyle, or even a direct effect on the brain (e.g. uraemia). As we have already noted, loss of sexual interest usually accompanies depression (p. 73).

Reactions of the partner

1. *Anxiety*: A partner may be worried about the effects of a disorder on sexual functioning, particularly where there has been no opportunity to discuss this with a member of the hospital team. Similar assumptions to those mentioned above may be held. The partner may believe that sexual activity will be impossible because of the disorder, or because of pain or physical damage that might result. This is more likely if the couple have difficulty in discussing their sexual relationship.

2. *Guilt.* A partner may feel guilty about sexual desires which conflict with concern felt about the partner's physical health. This may lead to avoidance of sexual activity and consequent resentment and friction.

The nature of the relationship

1. *Discord.* Although many couples find that physical illness in one of them brings them closer together, in others it results in alienation. There may be resentment about the changes in their respective roles which result from disability. The afflicted partner may be found unattractive because of bodily change or depression. Such reactions are more likely if the relationship has been unhappy prior to the onset of the disorder.

2. *Poor previous sexual adjustment.* If a couple's sexual relationship has been unsatisfactory prior to the physical disorder then sexual problems are more likely to occur. This may be because of

inhibitory attitudes towards sex which prevent adaptation to the disability, particularly if modification of sexual activity is necessary, or impaired communication which prevents expression of sexual needs and anxiety. The physical disability may be used by one or other partner as an excuse to avoid sex altogether.

Response of the medical profession

The ways in which the implications of physical illness and surgery are dealt with by medical personnel can determine subsequent sexual adjustment.
1. *Avoidance of discussion.* Discussion of sexual aspects of disease may be avoided because of embarrassment or lack of concern or information. Because of inadequate training in this aspect of medical care many doctors are unprepared to deal with topics concerning sexuality. They may adopt the policy of only providing information if a patient asks for it, and most patients are reluctant to do so. Alternatively, they may not be aware of the likely effects of physical illnesses on sexual performance, nor the psychological problems which commonly ensue. Lack of time may be given as a reason for the matter not being dealt with. However, advice about sexual activities can easily be incorporated into advice concerning other aspects of rehabilitation.
2. *Cursory discussion.* Superficial or general advice may be unhelpful because it will tend to leave patients to decide for themselves whether sexual activity will be possible in future and this decision may be based on ill-conceived notions about the effects of the illness.
3. *Inadequate information.* The sexual effects of many disorders and drugs, particularly in women, are poorly understood. Although an increasingly large body of information is available, many doctors feel inadequately equipped to give advice on sexual matters.

DRUGS

Prescribed drugs

A wide range of medication can affect sexual function (for reviews see Story 1974; Segraves 1977; *British Medical Journal* 1979;

Kolodny *et al.* 1979). Although it is rare for sexual side-effects to be assessed in controlled trials, occasionally a trial of treatment does yield valuable information about effects on sexuality. One notable example is the United Kingdom Medical Research Council trial of treatment of mild hypertension (*The Lancet* 1981). Comparison of the side-effects of bendrofluazide (a diuretic) and propranolol (an antihypertensive) with those of placebo drug treatment demonstrated that the two active drugs may both cause erectile dysfunction. In evaluating the possible sexual side-effects of many drugs one often has to rely on the somewhat unsatisfactory process of counting the number of published reports concerning each individual drug. The more important types of medication having sexual side-effects are listed at the end of this chapter in Table 5.5. It should be noted that none of them causes sexual problems in all patients. This raises the fascinating but unanswered question of why medication has adverse effects on the sexual functioning of some people and not of others. Presumably this reflects some form of physiological or pharmacological vulnerability.

The mechanism underlying sexual side-effects is often obscure. Some drugs appear to have direct effects on the brain, and these usually interfere with sexual interest, although the effect may be secondary to mood changes (e.g. methyldopa). Others interfere with the production or action of sex hormones. Probably the most common cause of sexual side-effects is interference with the autonomic nerve pathways involved in erectile response or ejaculation (e.g. tricyclic antidepressants, antihypertensives, and major tranquillizers).

In estimating the effects of medication on sexuality, account must also be taken of the likely effects of the physical condition for which it has been prescribed. For example, although antihypertensives undoubtedly can affect erectile function in many men, it is also known that men with untreated hypertension are more likely to have erectile problems than men with normal blood pressure (Bulpitt *et al.* 1976). Similarly, evaluation of the sexual side-effects of antidepressant medication is particularly difficult because of the serious effects that depression has on the sexual interest and performance of many men and women (Beaumont 1977; Mathew and Weinman 1982).

Two other widely used types of medication which *may* have

sexual side-effects should be mentioned. First, controversy still surrounds the possible effects of *oral contraception* on sexuality. Cartwright (1974) suggested that a quarter of women taking the pill had problems. A report by the Royal College of General Practitioners (1974) confirmed that more oral contraceptive users had impaired sexual interest than non-users, but also suggested that the effect was secondary to mood disturbance. Herzberg *et al.* (1971) found that after an initial increase in sexual interest and activity, pill users did not show the further increase in libido shown by women fitted with intrauterine devices. Some women either stopped taking or changed their pill, and in this group sexual interest was decreased. No significant hormonal abnormalities have been found in women on the pill who report sexual dysfunction compared with those without sexual difficulties (Bancroft *et al.* 1980). At present the most satisfactory conclusion is that oral contraception may affect sexual interest in some women, but the mechanism by which this occurs is obscure.

Secondly, several studies have demonstrated abnormalities of plasma sex hormone levels (LH and testosterone) and sex hormone binding globulin in both men and women on long-term *anticonvulsants*, especially phenytoin (Victor *et al.* 1977; Barragry *et al.* 1978; Toone *et al.* 1982). Anticonvulsants appear to cause an increase in sex hormone binding globulin, with a consequent reduction in free testosterone (although the *total* testosterone level as measured in routine blood tests will be raised). At present it is uncertain whether this finding contributes to the high percentage of patients with epilepsy who have sexual difficulties, including impaired sexual interest and erectile problems (Scott 1978).

Medication which may stimulate sexual interest or response. The age-old search for effective aphrodisiacs has not met with much success. A recent addition to the long list of putative aphrodisiacs is *amylnitrite*. This is a rapidly acting vasodilator which can intensify the experience of orgasm in both men and women. However, it can have cardiovascular side-effects and may cause headaches (Kolodny *et al.* 1979).

Androgens administered to men with normal serum testosterone levels do not appear to have any significant effects on sexual interest or potency, although they are beneficial in men with hypogonadal states (Davidson *et al.* 1979; Skakkebaek *et al.* 1981; Pirke and Kockott 1982).

Women who are given large doses of androgens have been noted to show an increase in sensitivity of the genitalia, response to sexual stimulation, and intensity of sexual gratification (Salmon and Geist 1943). This finding generated interest in the possible use of androgens in the treatment of women with impaired sexual interest. A study in which the effects of oral testosterone (Testoral) were compared with those of a minor tranquillizer (diazepam) appeared to lend support to the therapeutic use of androgens for this type of sexual dysfunction in women (Carney *et al.* 1978). However, further studies have not supported this finding (Mathews *et al.* 1983; Dow, personal communication). It seems likely that the positive effect of testosterone in the study by Carney and colleagues was an artefact resulting from the deleterious effect of the minor tranquillizer on sexual interest in the comparison group. The low dose and oral route of administration of the androgen used in these studies were such that circulating androgen levels were unlikely to be affected, but these were not investigated. An unpublished double-blind single-case study, by the author, of a woman with impaired sexual interest failed to reveal any change in blood androgen levels when she was on an oral preparation of testosterone compared with when she was receiving an inert placebo, and neither was there any improvement in her sexual interest.

Further work is required to investigate whether androgens have any role in the treatment of impaired sexual interest in women. It is possible that the dose of androgen required to have a significant effect on a woman's sexual interest will have unacceptable virilizing side-effects. It must also be remembered that impaired sexual interest very often results from psychological causes, especially problems in a couple's general relationship (p. 65), and even if androgens were to improve sexual interest it seems unlikely that drug treatment alone would be successful in such cases.

Non-prescribed drugs

Our knowledge about the effects on sexuality of non-prescribed drugs is surprisingly poor. This may be partly because of the difficulty of distinguishing specific drug effects from other non-specific effects which may result from drug use, such as debility, depression, and impaired interpersonal relationships. However, the information that is available suggests that some non-prescribed drugs may have profound effects on sexuality. Some of these drugs are considered below.

Alcohol, when used in moderate amounts, may reduce inhibitions and hence increase sexual arousal and interest. In assessing patients with sexual problems, especially impaired sexual interest, it is not uncommon to find that the dysfunction improves when an individual has been drinking. This may suggest that anxiety is contributing to the dysfunction. Alcohol primarily has a depressant effect on the central nervous system and in large amounts it therefore interferes with sexual arousal. In men this may cause erectile dysfunction, loss of pleasure, and retarded or absent ejaculation; impaired arousal and loss of pleasure and failure to reach orgasm are likely in women. The damaging effects of alcoholism on sexuality were discussed earlier (p. 74).

At present it is unclear whether *cigarette smoking* has effects on sexual function (Kolodny *et al.* 1979). Recent studies of small numbers of young men who smoked and who also suffered from erectile difficulties have suggested that cessation of smoking may lead to rapid reversal of the dysfunction (Forzberg *et al.* 1979; Forzberg and Olsson 1980). The link between smoking and arteriosclerosis, and the recognized effects of arteriosclerosis on erectile function (Wagner and Metz 1981), suggest that sexual dysfunction will be associated with prolonged heavy use of tobacco. This is an area for further research.

Although many *marihuana* users claim that the drug enhances their sexual experience, there is some evidence that in men it may have a deleterious effect on sexual response. There are conflicting reports concerning possible suppression of plasma testosterone levels with prolonged regular use of marihuana (Kolodny *et al.* 1974; Mendelson *et al.* 1974). However, some men who were chronic marihuana users and also had erectile dysfunction apparently experienced return of their potency within a few weeks of ceasing to use the drug (Kolodny *et al.* 1974). No negative effects of marihuana on female sexuality have yet been reported.

The effects of *opiates* (e.g. heroin and methadone) on sexual function are often profound. Impaired sexual interest, delayed ejaculation, and erectile failure have been reported in men (Cushman 1972), and impaired sexual interest in women (Gossop *et al.* 1974). Although these problems may reflect debility, depression, and the chaotic lifestyle of many addicts, hormonal disturbances may also be a factor. For example, various studies of men who were opiate addicts have demonstrated reduced plasma testosterone levels compared with those of non-drug users (e.g. Azizi *et al.* 1973; Cicero *et al.* 1975).

CONCLUSIONS

In this chapter the causes of sexual problems have been considered in some detail. One of the intriguing aspects of sexual medicine is its central position in relation to psychology, psychiatry, physical medicine, and pharmacology. Many patients who present at sexual dysfunction clinics have sexual problems resulting from factors in more than one of these areas. This emphasizes the need for therapists to keep an open mind with regard to aetiology in each case, and sometimes to tolerate considerable uncertainty about the relative importance of possible causal factors. In addition, this chapter should have made clear the necessity for sex therapists to ensure that they have a broad knowledge of the many causes of sexual problems, and the need for therapists working in non-medical settings to have easy access to specialist advice from general medicine, obstetrics and gynaecology, and psychiatry.

TABLE 5.3

Effects of physical illness on sexual function

System and disorder	Nature of the sexual problems	Comments
Cardiovascular		
Aortoiliac occlusive disease (blockage of the distal aorta, iliac, hypo-gastric or pudendal arteries)	Erectile dysfunction in 40-80% (Michal 1982)	Sexual function often improves after vascular surgery to remove the occlusion
Arteriosclerosis	Erectile dysfunction in 40-50% of men with evidence of peripheral vascular disease (Wagner & Metz 1981)	Often occurs in men with intermittent claudi-cation (calf pain on exercise). Arteriosclerosis may cause aortoiliac occlusion or restriction of peripheral vascular supply to the genitals
Hypertension	Erectile dysfunction and ejaculatory failure	Usually a side-effect of antihypertensive medication (p. 93), but erectile dysfunction may occur in untreated hypertensives
Myocardial infarction (heart attack)	*Men:* reduced sexual interest and activity (Tuttle *et al.* 1964; Bloch *et al.* 1975; Mehta & Krop 1979)	Often result of fear of relapse, angina, depression or lack of appropriate advice. May be related to concomitant hypertension, arteriosclerosis or drug treatment
Endocrine		
Adrenal insufficiency (Addison's disease)	*Women:* impaired sexual interest; reduced orgasmic capacity in some	Impaired sexual interest probably results from reduced androgen production
	Men: impaired sexual interest	Impaired sexual interest probably results from debility

TABLE 5.3 (*cont.*)

System and disorder	Nature of the sexual problems	Comments
Adrenal overactivity (Cushing's syndrome)	*Women:* variable effects on sexual interest; often unaffected, but may be increased or decreased in others. Orgasmic dysfunction in a few cases *Men:* diminished sexual interest in most cases; erectile dysfunction in the majority	Women may also experience virilism because of increased androgen production
Diabetes mellitus	*Men:* erectile dysfunction in approximately 50%; increasingly common with age, e.g. 23% aged 30-39 (McCulloch *et al.* 1980) and 75% aged 60-64 (Rubin & Babbott 1958). Retrograde ejaculation, ejaculatory failure and seepage of semen in a few cases *Women:* uncertainty about effects. Although orgasmic dysfunction has been reported (Kolodny 1971), recent studies suggest little effect on female sexuality, except reduced vaginal lubrication in some cases (Jensen 1981)	Male sexual dysfunction often appears to be result of peripheral neuropathy. Sexual dysfunction more likely where there is evidence of peripheral neuropathy and, or, bladder dysfunction. Cardiovascular abnormalities may be responsible in many cases. Psychological factors often appear important, usually as secondary reaction to early erectile difficulties (Fairburn *et al.* 1982). Transient erectile dysfunction can occur at times of poor diabetic control
Hypogonadism	*Men:* loss of sexual interest; erectile dysfunction and ejaculatory failure if hypogonadism severe	Examples of diseases: Klinefelter's syndrome, mumps orchitis, undescended testes, cirrhosis, and pituitary tumours. Dysfunction often

Women: natural menopause often associated with reduced sexual interest and orgasm, vaginal atrophy, and dyspareunia. Uncertain at present if complete removal of the ovaries has similar effects (Dennerstein & Burrows 1982)

reversed by testosterone administration (Davidson et al. 1979; Skakkebaek et al. 1981; Pirke & Kockott 1982)

Dysfunction usually reversed by hormone replacement therapy (Dennerstein & Burrows 1982)

Pituitary disease

Hyperprolactinaemia — Erectile dysfunction

Hyperprolactinaemia may be caused by e.g. pituitary adenoma, phenothiazine medication. If sexual dysfunction present there is usually abnormally low plasma testosterone level. Dysfunction often reversed by administration of bromocriptine (Thorner & Besser 1977)

Hypopituitarism — *Men*: impaired sexual interest; erectile dysfunction, and ejaculatory failure

Women: impaired sexual interest and orgasmic dysfunction in most cases

Sexual dysfunction results from hypogonadotrophic hypogonadism

Thyroid disease

Hyperthyroidism (thyrotoxicosis) — *Men*: occasionally hypersexuality, more often unaltered or impaired sexual interest. Erectile dysfunction common

Women: most cases unaffected. Occasional hypersexuality or impaired sexual interest

Dysfunction corrected by treatment of hyperthyroidism

TABLE 5.3 (cont.)

System and disorder	Nature of the sexual problems	Comments
Hypothyroidism	Men: impaired sexual interest in majority; erectile dysfunction in some	Effects probably result partly from debility, and partly from reduced synthesis of testosterone and abnormal metabolism of androgens and oestrogens. Dysfunction reversed with appropriate treatment of hypothyroidism.
	Women: impaired sexual interest in majority; orgasmic dysfunction in some (Kolodny et al. 1979)	
Genito-urinary: men		
Peyronie's disease (curvature of penis because of fibrosis)	Often erectile dysfunction or painful erections	Usually irreversible
Priapism (unrelieved erection in absence of sexual stimulation)	Erectile dysfunction	May be associated with e.g. malignancy, blood dyscrasia, or anticoagulant therapy. Often no apparent cause. Usually irreversible
Prostatitis	Painful ejaculation in some cases. Occasionally pain on erection	Pain may be located in rectum, testes or glans penis
Urethritis	Occasionally causes pain on ejaculation	
Venereal disease	Rarely a direct cause of sexual dysfunction, except pain on ejaculation	Sexual dysfunction found in quarter of men with venereal disease (Catalan el al. 1981; p. 51). Presumed aetiology psychological
Genito-urinary: women		
Clitoral adhesions	Uncertain	
Imperforate hymen	Dyspareunia and vaginismus	

Pelvic inflammatory disease (infection or endometriosis)	Deep dyspareunia
Vaginitis (because of infection/oestrogen insufficiency)	Dyspareunia (burning pain)
Venereal disease	Rarely a direct cause of sexual dysfunction, except dyspareunia. Sexual dysfunction found in two-fifths of women with venereal disease (Catalan *et al.* 1981; p. 51). Presumed aetiology psychological
Musculo-skeletal	
Arthritis	Mechanical difficultis and pain impeding sexual intercourse and caressing. Impaired sexual interest because of fatigue. In Sjogren's syndrome may be impaired vaginal lubrication and dyspareunia
Neurological	
Epilepsy	Impaired sexual interest often reported (Scott 1978, especially in patients with temporal lobe epilepsy (Taylor 1969). Anticonvulsants may have effects on sexuality (p. 81)
Strokes	*Men*: erectile capacity and sexual interest usually soon restored. Approximately half do not resume sexual relationships (Hawton 1984). Dominant hemisphere lesions may often cause impaired sexual interest (Kalliomaki *et al.* 1961). Sexual difficulties usually psychological in origin
Other focal brain	Frontal lobe lesions can cause disinhibition
Spinal cord transection	*Men*: complete lesions cause erectile dysfunction and failure of ejaculation—may be reflex erections. Effects of partial lesions depend. Psychological reactions to paraplegia/tetraplegia likely to increase sexual difficulties (Silver & Owens 1975)

TABLE 5.3 (*cont.*)

System and disorder	Nature of the sexual problems	Comments
	on site of lesion—ejaculation usually affected by lesions at any level, especially lower lesions; erection often retained in high lesions (Higgins 1978)	
	Women: orgasmic dysfunction if complete cord lesion (Higgins 1978)	
Multiple sclerosis	Depends on severity of disorder. *Men:* erectile dysfunction (often partial) in 43% (Vas 1978) to 62% (Lilius *et al.* 1976; Lundberg 1980)	Dysfunction probably result of involvement of lateral horns of spinal cord in disease process (Vas 1978). Impaired sensation in genital region and testicular atrophy may occur. Psychological factors often important
Peripheral nerves		
Neuropathy (e.g. diabetic, alcoholic)	*See* diabetes mellitus	
Renal		
Renal failure and dialysis	*Men:* erectile difficulties and impaired sexual interest common both in chronic renal failure and renal dialysis (Abram *et al.* 1975)	Causes unknown. Psychological factors, electrolyte and hormonal abnormalties have all been implicated
	Women: impaired sexual interest common (Steele *et al.* 1976)	
Respiratory		
Chronic obstructive airways disease (chronic bronchitis, emphysema and asthma)	Impaired ability to participate in or enjoy sexual activity because of respiratory distress	

TABLE 5.4.
Effects of surgery on sexual function

Type of surgery	*Nature of sexual problems*	*Comment*
Gastro-intestinal		
Intestinal stomas (e.g. colostomy)	See below	Where rectal surgery (see below) has not been involved, the stoma may affect sexuality because of embarrassment and sense of unattractiveness
Rectal resection	*Men*: erectile dysfunction and ejaculatory difficulties often occur, although less common with modern techniques	Caused by damage to pelvic nerves
	Women: some develop dyspareunia. (Burnham *et al*. 1976)	
Genito-urinary		
Prostatectomy	Often causes retrograde ejaculation. Radical perineal prostatectomy usually causes erectile dysfunction because of damage to pelvic nerves	Sexual dysfunction may occur for psychological reasons after prostatectomy for benign conditions
Gynaecological		
Episiotomy	Often causes dyspareunia; may be long-lasting in a few cases	

TABLE 5.4 (cont.)

Type of surgery	Nature of sexual problems	Comment
Hysterectomy	Rarely causes sexual dysfunction; often leads to improved sexual adjustment	Although several authors have claimed that hysterectomy leads to sexual dysfunction in many women, prospective research has not supported this claim (e.g. Gath et al. 1982)
Wertheim's hysterectomy for carcinoma of uterus	Restriction of length of vagina, precluding deep penetration	
Oophorectomy (removal of ovaries)	? Reduced sexual interest and orgasm, and vaginal atrophy and dyspareunia	See Table 5.3—hypogonadism
Vaginal repair of prolapse	Dyspareunia in some cases	More likely with posterior repair (Francis & Jeffcoate 1961)
Amputation	Mechanical difficulties may rule out use of some positions for sexual intercourse. Phantom limb sensations and tender stump may interfere with enjoyment of sexual activity	Psychological factors concerning body image also likely to be important
Mastectomy	Sexual dysfunction (cessation of sexual intercourse or failure to enjoy it) in one-third a year after operation. (Maguire et al. 1978)	Difficulties likely to result from sense of unattractiveness, depression, or revulsion on part of partner

TABLE 5.5

Effects of medication on sexual function

Medication	Possible effects on sexual function		
	Interest	*Arousal*	*Orgasm*
Anticholingergic			
Probanthine		Erectile dysfunction	
Antidepressants			
Tricyclics	Reduced	Erectile dysfunction	Retarded ejaculation; delayed or absent orgasm (women)
MAOIs		Erectile dysfunction	Retarded ejaculation; delayed or absent orgasm (women)
Lithium carbonate	Reduced	Erectile dysfunction	
Antihypertensives			
(1) Central acting: methyldopa	Reduced	Erectile dysfunction	Retarded ejaculation
(2) Ganglion blockers: Hexamethonium Mecamylamine		Erectile dysfunction	Failure of ejaculation or retrograde ejaculation
(3) Alpha-blockers: Indoramin			Failure of ejaculation
(4) Beta-blockers: Propranolol	Reduced	Erectile dysfunction	

TABLE 5.5 (*cont.*)

Medication	Possible effects on sexual function		
	Interest	*Arousal*	*Orgasm*
(5) Adrenergic blockers:			
Guanethidine	Reduced	Erectile dysfunction	Failure of ejaculation or retrograde ejaculation
Bethanidine			
Diuretics			
(1) Thiazides:			
Bendrofluazide		Erectile dysfunction	
(2) Spironolactone	Reduced (may also cause gynaecomastia)	Erectile dysfunction	
Hormones			
(1) Corticosteroids	Reduced	Erectile dysfunction	Retarded ejaculation
(2) Oestrogens	Reduced (men)	Erectile dysfunction	Retarded ejaculation
Hypnotics			
Barbiturates	Reduced	Erectile dysfunction	Retarded ejaculation
Major tranquillizers			
(1) Phenothiazines:			
Thioridazine	Reduced	Erectile dysfunction	Retarded or absent ejaculation (often)
Chlorpromazine	Reduced	Erectile dysfunction	
(2) Butyrophenones:			
Haloperidol		Erectile dysfunction	

Part II

Management of sexual problems

In Part I, sexual problems were considered in terms of the types of problems for which people seek help, their prevalence in the general population, their effects on people's lives, and their causes. With this information to hand, together with the introduction to sexual anatomy and sexual response provided in Chapter 2, we can now turn our attention to the principal focus of this book, namely how sexual problems can be alleviated. This section includes enough detail to serve as a practical manual for therapists. However, the written word may not be sufficient by itself; anyone wishing to gain practical experience in sex therapy should also try to obtain supervision from an experienced therapist.

Chapters 6-13 concern the treatment of couples. Before initiating sex therapy a careful assessment must be carried out. This is described step-by-step in Chapter 6, together with general guidelines and an indication of the types of patients suitable for sex therapy. Once a couple have been accepted for treatment, the programme is introduced by providing them with a formulation of their problem, including a brief outline of likely causes. This procedure is described and illustrated in Chapter 7.

The rest of treatment consists of three essential components. The first comprises the homework assignments which are central to sex therapy (Chapter 8). These have the function of providing a couple with a graduated programme for rebuilding their sexual relationship and bringing to the fore factors which are contributing to the sexual problem. Secondly, there are the extremely important general aspects of the relationship between the therapist and a couple and the techniques that are available to help a couple when they encounter difficulties with the homework assignments. The skills of an experienced psychotherapist are not essential. However, the therapist should be able to form a warm and trusting relationship with couples. Equally, the therapist must have sufficient psychological awareness to be able to help couples when they encounter difficulties during therapy. These aspects of sex therapy are discussed in Chapter 9. The third component of the programme is educational (Chapter 10). Sexual information can usefully be provided by devoting a part of therapy specifically to this purpose, and by recommending appropriate reading material. General relationship issues often become apparent during sex therapy. Means of helping with these, using the same principles as are employed in sex therapy, are discussed in Chapter 11.

How treatment ends can be just as important as how it begins. The process of ending treatment, good and bad outcome, and ways of obtaining standardized outcome assessments, are described in Chapter 12. In Chapter 13, the findings of research investigations into the application and outcome of sex therapy with couples are critically examined.

When this type of treatment was first introduced it appeared to offer little to people without partners. Fortunately, this situation has changed considerably, and in Chapter 14 are described treatment approaches for individuals with sexual problems. Also in that chapter are considered treatment in groups, brief counselling, and how people may be helped to cope with sexual problems resulting from physical disorders.

The book ends with an overview of the place of sex therapy today, and consideration of important clinical and research needs in this field.

6

Assessment

Before entering sex therapy a couple must be carefully assessed. This should enable the therapist to establish whether or not they are likely to benefit from treatment. In addition it should allow some understanding of how and why their sexual problems developed, although the precise origins of the problem are often unclear at this stage and can only be clarified during treatment. As the assessment proceeds, the therapist should form some initial hypotheses about likely causal factors and how these will influence the partners' approaches to the homework assignments.

We will first consider which couples are likely to respond to sex therapy. Then the aims and general features of the assessment procedure will be examined. The rest of the chapter is devoted to detailed consideration of the areas which should be covered during the assessment. Checklists of these are provided in tables at the end of this chapter.

SUITABILITY FOR SEX THERAPY

There are no absolute guidelines concerning which couples are suitable for sex therapy and which are unlikely to respond, and prediction of outcome is often difficult (p. 205). The following are some of the important factors to be considered in assessing suitability:

Nature of the sexual problem

First, it should be established that the couple actually have a sexual dysfunction, or are markedly dissatisfied with their sexual relationship in some clearly defined way. The reason for seeking help may be because of misunderstanding or unreasonable expectations about sexuality. Secondly, before offering treatment, the therapist should be clear about the precise nature of the couple's sexual difficulty. Sometimes, in spite of careful assessment, a couple remain vague about the problem. This may disguise the fact that their problem is not primarily sexual, but of a more general nature.

General relationship

A couple whose sexual problem is the result of major difficulties in their general relationship are unlikely to be suitable for sex therapy, at least in the first instance. When the therapist is uncertain which type of difficulty is paramount this should be made clear to the couple. It is sometimes appropriate to offer a limited trial of treatment, say three sessions, with an understanding that at the end of this trial period the therapist will help the couple examine their progress and decide whether to continue with sex therapy. A couple whose relationship is characterized by chronic resentment and hostility, with a lack of affection or love on one or both sides, are extremely unlikely to benefit from sex therapy.

It is unwise to begin sex therapy with a couple when one partner is known to be having an affair. An unfaithful partner is unlikely to direct his or her full attention to the treatment programme, and jealousy and resentment may prevent the other partner from benefiting. In any case, infidelity may reflect general instability in the relationship. The couple might be offered treatment if the therapist feels optimistic about the outcome of therapy, provided the affair is ended.

Motivation

If the motivation of either or both partners seems poor, sex therapy is unlikely to be successful. However, one partner may appear to be poorly motivated because of lack of understanding of his or her role in helping the dysfunctional partner to get over the problem. In such circumstances, if it is clear to the therapist that couple rather than individual treatment is needed, the couple should be encouraged to have a trial of three or four sessions of treatment. The attitude of a resistant partner may change fairly quickly, especially if it soon becomes clear that not only is the problem likely to improve, but that the sexual relationship is becoming generally more rewarding.

Sometimes, one or both partners say they want help, and superficially appear well-motivated, but have not appreciated the full implication of entering sex therapy. The extent of their motivation will become apparent once treatment begins.

Psychiatric disorder

Severe psychiatric disorder in either partner precludes immediate sex therapy. *Depression* is the most common disorder encountered in couples seeking help for sexual problems. The term 'depression' here does not just mean unhappiness, but the type of disorder which might itself require treatment. If this is the case, sex therapy should be postponed until the condition has resolved. Depression is a common cause of sexual difficulties, especially impaired sexual interest (p. 73). In such cases, treatment directed more specifically at the depression or its causes would be appropriate. However, mild depression or anxiety are common reactions to sexual difficulties, and a couple should not be excluded from sex therapy because of this.

Serious and continuing *alcohol abuse* in either partner would also preclude sex therapy. If acceptable to the couple, referral for help with the drinking problem would be indicated in the first instance. Sex therapy should only be considered again after a reasonable period of abstinence.

It is more difficult to provide guidelines concerning how other neurotic and personality problems affect suitability for sex therapy. People with severe *anxiety states* often find difficulty in engaging in the homework assignments, but may benefit sufficiently from anxiety management techniques that later involvement is possible. People with *obsessional symptoms or traits*, provided these are not too severe, can often benefit from sex therapy.

Physical illness

Physical illness does not preclude treatment. In fact, helping couples with sexual dysfunction resulting from physical disorders (e.g. diabetes mellitus, multiple sclerosis) is often relatively easy, although the gaols of treatment may differ from those with able-bodied couples (p. 238). Sex therapy should not be offered, however, until any physical causes of the sexual problem have been fully investigated and treated appropriately. Similarly, when sexual dysfunction is the result of drug treatment, the first step is to ascertain whether there is any alternative medication which interferes less with sexual function.

Pregnancy

Pregnancy usually affects sexual interest, especially during the third trimester. It is unwise, therefore, to begin sex therapy if the woman is pregnant, however early the pregnancy. Furthermore, the pregnancy may provide a plausible excuse for lack of progress. The couple should be reassessed some three to six months after the birth because by then, under normal circumstances, sexual interest should largely have returned.

Although not essential, fertile couples should be strongly advised to use contraception during treatment, even if they are keen on having a pregnancy. Any anxiety about conception, and the possible deleterious effects of early pregnancy, can then be avoided until treatment is completed.

AIMS OF ASSESSMENT

The assessment of couples for sex therapy has several purposes in addition to determining suitability. First, by detailed questioning the therapist should be able to identify the precise nature and development of the couple's problems. This should allow the aims of therapy to be established, including the target problem and the changes which each partner would like to achieve.

Secondly, careful enquiry about each partner's background, including sexual development, and sexual attitudes and information, should allow the therapist to develop at least some understanding of the causes of the problem. This provides information that can be used in the formulation of the problem with the couple (Chapter 7).

Thirdly, the interaction between the therapist and the partners at this stage is part of the therapeutic process. For example, by asking questions about sexuality in a calm, reassuring manner the therapist can alleviate a couple's anxieties and demonstrate that frank discussion of sexuality is feasible. The therapist may provide sexual information during the assessment in response to anxieties expressed about some form of sexual behaviour, such as masturbation, or to dispel fears and mistaken beliefs. Finally, the therapist may clarify a problem which was previously regarded by a couple as obscure, permanent, and a source of shame, bewilderment, and distress, and this can prove highly therapeutic.

GENERAL ASPECTS OF THE ASSESSMENT

Before beginning the assessment, the therapist should explain its aims to both partners together. Following this introduction the partners should *always* then be interviewed separately. This allows each partner an equal opportunity to express his or her views on the problem. It also provides an opportunity for disclosure of personal information which has never been discussed with the partner. This might, for example, have particular relevance to the couple's suitability for treatment (e.g. information concerning a current affair), or to the therapist's understanding of the problem (e.g. guilt about masturbation in a man with premature ejaculation). To encourage disclosure of such information each partner should be reassured about the confidentiality of the interview, and especially that the therapist will respect their wishes not to reveal to the partner anything they do not wish to be known (p. 104).

For the therapist who is working singly it is usually best to interview first the partner who sought help. If both partners sought help then they might themselves decide who should be interviewed first. Co-therapists often adopt the policy of each therapist taking a detailed history from the same-sex partner, and then, during the second interview, only briefly assessing the other partner's attitudes and reactions to the sexual problem.

At the beginning of each assessment interview the therapist should indicate how much time is available in order that the partners do not feel unduly rushed and can anticipate the pace of the interview. For a thorough assessment, usually about three-quarters of an hour to one hour is required with each partner. The therapist might find it convenient to conduct the two interviews on separate occasions.

Note-taking

The therapist will need to take notes, but the necessity for this should be explained, namely to serve as a reminder at a later date. The partners should be reassured about the confidentiality of the notes (p. 156). It is best not to take detailed notes at the beginning of the interview, but to give the person one's full attention, listening to what is being said about the nature and development of the problem, asking appropriate questions to encourage a full account, and, as is often necessary at this stage, providing reassurance if the person becomes distressed or appears embarrassed. Once a clear picture of the presenting problem has been established, the therapist can summarize this, and then record the summary in the notes. For other aspects of the assessment (such as family history, medical history, etc.), it is usually more appropriate to take notes while asking questions.

Nature of the questions

The assessment interview should not be like an inquisition in which the therapist fires questions one after another. Generally, it is worth beginning with relatively non-embarrassing questions before asking for sexually explicit information. This will allow the person more chance to develop confidence in the therapist. If the person becomes very embarrassed when being asked about a particularly sensitive topic it is best to move to less threatening questions and then to return later to this area. The therapist might also acknowledge the person's embarrassment by explaining that many people find it difficult to talk about such intimate matters but that this gradually becomes easier. However, it is essential not to avoid issues because they are embarrassing—they may well be central to the couple's problem.

Whenever possible the therapist should begin by using *open-ended questions* in order to obtain as much spontaneous information as possible, in the person's own words. These include questions such as 'Tell me how the problem began' and 'How did your husband's problem affect you?'. Later, *closed or direct questions* can be asked in order to complete the picture. These include questions such as 'Did you ever feel guilty about masturbation?', and 'Have you ever had a climax?'. A direct question might be preceded by a reflective summary. For example, 'I think you are saying that when lovemaking is getting to the point where you think about intercourse, you immediately wonder whether you will be able to keep your erection long enough, you start to become anxious, and it is then you feel your erection going. Is that how it happens?'. Closed questions can be useful when a person is becoming embarrassed because they can relieve the person of some of the burden of using difficult vocabulary.

The type of vocabulary that is used during assessment interviews (and in subsequent therapy) is very important. Many couples will not be familiar with medical terms, and the therapist may feel uncomfortable using colloquial expressions which may be more familiar to the patient. In addition, colloquial terms are often imprecise, and couples may be uncomfortable using them in a clinical setting. The therapist must find out what terms the partners understand, and then try to reach some common ground over the vocabulary to be used in the future. Some terms, such as 'to come', describing either a man's ejaculation or a woman's orgasm, are almost universally used by lay people and can usefully be employed in treatment.

The inexperienced therapist may feel embarrassed and uncomfortable when beginning to take sexual histories. This is understandable, particularly in view of the paucity of attention paid in many professional training courses to the topic of human sexuality. However, ease about such interviewing usually develops rapidly with practice and the resulting confidence experienced by the therapist is likely to be reassuring for couples. Role-playing interviews with other trainees or an experienced therapist is one way of gaining such confidence.

In order to clarify the nature of the problem, the couple should be asked to provide a detailed account of a specific occasion on which difficulty was experienced. This is more informative than a general description of the problem. The account should include not only what happened, but what each person was thinking and feeling, and what he or she thought the partner was thinking and feeling. This detailed account of a single episode is best obtained later in the interview when the person is more relaxed.

It is also important that the therapist remembers at the end of each interview to ask if anything has been discussed which should not be revealed to the partner. If information about a current affair has been revealed the therapist will have to explain that this precludes sex therapy for the present. Should a partner have revealed some other confidential information which might be important in treatment (e.g. a long history of faking orgasm), the therapist must agree to the person's request to keep this from the partner. However, the therapist should explain that if it becomes apparent during treatment that sharing this information with the partner is necessary in order for progress to occur, this will be discussed again outside a conjoint session.

Conjoint assessment

After interviewing both partners separately the therapist should then see them together again. If there was some important discrepancy between their individual accounts of the problem, this conjoint interview allows the therapist to explore this further, and, hopefully, to clarify it. However, the main purpose in seeing the partners together is to gain an impression of how they relate to each other. The therapist can assess how they discuss sexuality; whether they appear supportive of each other; and whether one partner views the other as having the sexual problem, or whether they share responsibility for the problem.

Finally, the therapist should explain the conclusions that he or she has reached concerning further management. This includes the couple's suitability for sex therapy, or, for example, indications for marital therapy or physical investigations.

Cultural problems

An increasingly important issue concerns the management of couples from different cultural backgrounds from that of the therapist, especially those from other ethnic groups. Some understanding of the sexual values of the particular culture is usually essential. For example, many Asian men find totally unacceptable the suggestion that their partners should have an equal opportunity to initiate sexual activity. In such situations, therapists are advised to find, or supervise, another therapist who is familiar with the sexual values of the particular culture. Should this prove impossible, the therapist should explain the difficulty to the couple and then try to help them, modifying the sex therapy programme in whatever way is necessary to accommodate their value system. In spite of these cross-cultural difficulties, sex therapy can be applied with reasonable success in clinics dealing with mixed racial communities (Christopher 1982).

ASSESSMENT SCHEDULE

The details of an assessment schedule that has been found useful in clinical practice are given below. In working through such a schedule, one should not simply ask a long series of questions and record the answers; the information should be organized in the therapist's mind in order to establish a clear picture of each partner and the relationship. Apart from clarifying the precise nature of the presenting problem, the therapist should also try to identify any factors in the partners' backgrounds which might have predisposed them to develop a sexual problem later in life, possible precipitants for the problem, and factors which may be maintaining it. If, at the end of the assessment, it is difficult to put together a formulation of the problem, the therapist should consider whether any important questions have been omitted, or whether there has been any misunderstanding. However, while the assessment should be thorough, in many instances important aspects of the aetiology will for the present remain obscure. Important causal factors which have not yet been revealed will often become apparent during therapy, although successful therapy may occur without the full aetiology ever being revealed.

The assessment schedule is summarized in Table 6.1 at the end of this chapter and discussed in detail below. For the sake of clarity this is largely in note form.

1. *The nature and development of the sexual problem*

This includes detailed clarification of the nature of the problem (or problems), including when and how it began, how it subsequently developed, any factors that have made it worse (e.g. stress at work, general disharmony, medication), and any that have led to improvement (e.g. alcohol, holidays, use of erotic literature). The therapist should establish what have been the effects of the problem on both partners.

In order to identify any remaining difficulties, the therapist should enquire specifically about *sexual interest, arousal,* and *orgasm* or *ejaculation.*

The following are some further questions the therapist should try to answer about particular problems once the broad category of problem presented by the couple has been identified:

(i) *Impaired sexual interest.*
Is loss of interest in sex with the partner complete, or is the person sometimes interested?

Is the problem only partner-related, or is it total? Thus, do sexual day-dreams, masturbation, or sexual attraction to other people occur?

Is this an isolated problem or has it been accompanied by other symptoms, either physical (e.g. lack of energy) or psychological (e.g. depression)?

Has the problem accompanied other changes in the relationship between the partners (e.g. loss of affection, impaired communication, rows)?

(ii) *Orgasmic dysfunction.*
Does orgasm occur under any circumstances—during sexual intercourse, with manual stimulation, during oral sex, during masturbation, during sleep?

Does the woman get aroused?

Does she think she receives enough or appropriate stimulation from her partner?

Does she ever feel close to orgasm?

Does high arousal evoke anxiety?

Does the woman use sexual fantasies?

If a woman is unsure whether she ever has an orgasm the therapist should ask her to describe her experience. An account suggesting increasing arousal, with tension reaching a peak and then being released, possibly accompanied by a sense of fulfilment and relaxation, suggests she is orgasmic. If, in response to specific questioning, she describes the experience of regular vaginal muscle contractions in association with such an experience, this confirms that she is orgasmic. However, some women do not feel these muscle contractions (even if demonstrated by physiological investigation in a laboratory).

(iii) *Vaginismus.*
Do attempts at penetration evoke pain?
Where does the pain occur?
Does the pain occur even if the woman is aroused?
Is the woman (or her partner) aware of spasm of the vaginal muscles?
Is vaginal penetration ever possible?
Has vaginal examination by a doctor caused a similar experience to attempts at sexual intercourse?
Can the woman use tampons?
Has she, or her partner, ever tried inserting a finger into her vagina, and was this possible?

(iv) *Dyspareunia* (female).
Where does the pain occur (at the entrance to, or deep in, the vagina)?
What type of pain is it (e.g. sharp and stinging, or dull ache)?
Does the woman also get pain in her back?
Does she ever experience pain on passing water?
Is there any evidence of vaginal infection (discharge, itching)?
Has there been any vaginal trauma (rape, childbirth)?
Does she experience the pain even if sexually aroused?

(v) *Erectile dysfunction.*
Can the man get an erection under any circumstances at all?
Is the erection full or partial? (corroborative information from the man's partner will be important because the man may underestimate his erection).
Are there any abnormalities in the shape of the erection?
Does he get an erection during sexual activity and then lose it at a particular point (e.g. just before or just after vaginal penetration)?
Can he get an erection on his own (e.g. during masturbation, or when having erotic fantasies), and can he keep it if he wishes?
Does he ever wake up at night with an erection, or have an erection on waking in the morning?

(vi) *Premature ejaculation.*
When does ejaculation occur (e.g. before vaginal penetration, immediately after beginning sexual intercourse)?
Is it pleasurable?
Has the delay between insertion and ejaculation shortened?
Does anything help delay ejaculation (e.g. alcohol, distracting thoughts, frequent sexual intercourse)?
Does anything make the problem worse (e.g. tiredness, short or long foreplay)?

Does or did the man masturbate rapidly?
Was guilt associated with masturbation?

(vii) *Retarded ejaculation.*
Can the man ejaculate under any circumstances (with his partner, during masturbation, in his sleep)?
If not, has he ever been able to ejaculate?
Is ejaculation pleasurable?

2. Family background and early childhood

Parents' and siblings' ages. Family deaths and dates of deaths. Nature of parents' relationship, including whether they appeared to show each other affection.
Childhood: happy and unhappy aspects. Nature and closeness of relationships with parents; was affection received from them? Nature of relationships with siblings.
Attitudes of family to sex. Was sex discussed in the home? If so, in what context and what impression did this have on the patient?
Family history of physical illness (e.g. diabetes) and of psychiatric disorder.

3. Early sexual development and experience

Age of puberty (development of secondary sexual characteristics). Was this about average for the person's peer group, or did he or she develop earlier or later than peers? If earlier, or later, did this cause embarrassment, anxiety, or sense of inferiority? General attitudes to early sexual development.
For female partner: age of menarche; had she received prior information? Reaction to first menstruation.
Any upsetting sexual experiences that occurred during childhood.
Age at which first developed sexual interest in opposite sex.
Masturbation. Ask 'when did you find out about masturbation?' This allows people to tell you when they began to masturbate, or, if they have not, when they first heard about it. Attitudes to masturbation.
Age at which had first boyfriend/girlfriend. Nature of early relationships with opposite sex. Age when had first sexual

experience (if before met current partner). Nature of this experience and attitude towards it.

Subsequent heterosexual relationships: the nature of these and whether there were any problems in either the general or sexual aspects of the relationships.

Any history of homosexual interest/behaviour. Has such interest/behaviour persisted, or was it a transient (e.g. adolescent) phase?

4. *Sexual information*

Source of sexual information (parents, friends, jokes, books, experience).

Does person think that knowledge about sexuality is adequate? (The therapist should also make an assessment of the person's level of sexual knowledge on the basis of responses to questions throughout the interview.)

5. *Current relationship*

When and how met partner. What attracted person to partner? How relationship developed.

Sexual relationship: when first began. How it developed. Was it at any time satisfying to the person/were there problems early on and, if so, what were they? Effect of marriage on sexual relationship (if began before marriage). Partners' ability to communicate about sex.

General relationship: affection, friction, interest, social activities, friends, communication. Effect of marriage on general relationship.

Children: ages, effects of pregnancy and childbirth on sexual relationship. Nature of relationship with children and attitudes to their sexuality.

What form of contraception, if any, is being used? Attitudes to future contraception.

Infidelity: any affairs during this relationship? Have there been problems in other sexual relationships? Is there a current affair?

Commitment: how committed is the person to this relationship? Any thoughts of separation? Likely consequences if sexual problem persists?

6. *Schooling and occupations*

Brief account of schooling, achievements, and occupations. Details of current occupation. Is it particularly stressful or tiring? Is it satisfying? For housewives: how demanding is housework; any help available?

7. *Interests*

Hobbies and interests. Are these shared with partner?

8. *Religious beliefs*

Has the person ever held strong religious beliefs? Do these affect the person's attitudes to sexuality? Are religious beliefs shared by both partners?

9. *Medical history*

Nature of any past/current illnesses/operations.
(For women) any problems with menstruation?
Current and recent medication.

10. *Psychiatric history*

Nature of any past/current psychiatric disorder and its treatment.

11. *Use of alcohol and drugs (including smoking)*

12. *Appearance and mood (i.e. mental state)*

It is rarely necessary to carry out a formal examination of mental state as is often done in psychiatric assessments. However, the therapist should assess each partner's appearance and mood throughout the interview. In particular, the therapist should look for signs suggesting depression (e.g. sad or dishevelled appearance, crying, pessimism) or anxiety (persistent apprehension, trembling, pallor, hesitations). If there is any suspicion of such disorder the therapist must enquire specifically about the person's mood, sleeping pattern, appetite and weight, energy, concentration, and memory. If the person is depressed, the therapist should always ask about attitudes to the future, and suicidal ideas.

A full psychiatric assessment must be carried out if it appears that the person has a moderate or severe psychiatric disorder. If the therapist is not appropriately qualified to do this, a psychiatric opinion should be sought.

13. *Goals and motivation*

At the end of the assessment interview with each partner the therapist should try to establish the precise changes in both the sexual and general relationship the person would like to achieve through treatment. Accurate assessment of motivation is often difficult as it may only become fully apparent once treatment begins. Nevertheless, the therapist must assess each partner's motivation as far as is possible. This includes determining to what extent responsibility for the problem is shared, who sought help, the consequences of any previous attempts at solving the problem (either with assistance or through self-help), and the couple's primary goal in seeking help. Couples who seek help with fertility problems (e.g. non-consummation, retarded ejaculation) and for whom conception is the only goal are often very difficult to help.

14. *Physical examination and investigation*

In some sex therapy clinics a physical and sexual examination of both partners is carried out routinely for both diagnostic and therapeutic purposes. This is inappropriate in non-medical settings and is in any case often unnecessary. Because of the highly intrusive nature of such a procedure when there is no obvious indication for it, a physical examination of this kind is probably best restricted to those partners for whom it may be therapeutic, and those whose histories suggest the possibility of an undetected physical cause for their problem. Women with vaginismus, and people with anxieties about the size, shape or some other characteristics of their genitals are examples of the first category. A physical examination for diagnostic purposes is indicated for men with erectile dysfunction and women with dyspareunia, and is appropriate for some people with impaired sexual interest.

If necessary, the physical examination may be carried out after the assessment interviews, provided the therapist is appropriately qualified. Sometimes, as in the case of vaginismus (p. 143), the examination may be incorporated later in the treatment programme. However, non-medical therapists, and medical therapists not wishing to do physical examinations in this setting, should request that either the person's family doctor, or another physician, performs the examination if one is necessary.

In addition, blood tests, or a special investigation, may be indicated. However, the special investigations (see below) are available in very few centres in the UK.

Men. A summary of key aspects of the physical examination and of some of the investigations that may be indicated in men is presented in Table 6.2 at the end of this chapter.

The physical examination should begin with a search for general signs of illness. Hair distribution and breast development should be studied for any indication of hormonal disturbance. Because of the various ways in which disorders of the cardiovascular system can affect sexuality (Chapter 5), a thorough check should be carried out, but particular attention should be paid to the man's blood pressure and peripheral pulses. A marked fall of blood pressure upon standing up can be a sign of damage to the autonomic nervous system. Examination of the deep reflexes and sensation in the lower limbs will also assist in the detection of peripheral neuropathy.

The important aspects of the genital examination are listed in Table 6.2. Testicular sensation is tested by applying firm pressure to each testicle in turn. A normal response is the experience of discomfort with moderate pressure. Reduced or absent testicular sensation is often found with other signs of autonomic neuropathy, as in diabetic neuropathy (Campbell *et al.* 1974).

Blood tests for sex hormone levels are indicated in all men with erectile dysfunction when the problem is not clearly situational, and in men with impaired sexual interest or ejaculatory failure. A testosterone level will identify hypogonadism. The LH level will help distinguish hypergonadotropic (primary testicular failure) from hypogonadotropic hypogonadism (secondary testicular failure). A blood test for fasting glucose should also be carried out in all cases of non-situational erectile dysfunction. If this is abnormal, or if diabetes is strongly suspected, a glucose tolerance test is indicated. If the man's testosterone level is abnormally low a prolactin level should be obtained to test for hyperprolactinaemia. When retrograde ejaculation is suspected the man should be asked to save a sample of post-coital urine. If he is ejaculating into his bladder the sample may appear cloudy and sperms will be visible under a microscope.

The special investigations listed in Table 6.2 are largely unavailable to most sex therapists in the UK, but may become more widely available in future as they are currently in the USA. However, the vast majority of sexual disorders with a physical basis can be diagnosed from the history of the problem, or from either a physical examination or blood tests. The rest should become apparent early in sex therapy, although the precise cause may not be clear without further investigation.

Nocturnal erections are normally associated with dream or rapid-eye movement (REM) sleep. Simultaneous recordings of penile tumescence, using a special strain gauge, and of the sleeping EEG, have been used to differentiate psychogenic from organic erectile dysfunction. However, this method is not entirely reliable (Fisher *et al.* 1978), and usually necessitates the man spending at least one night in a laboratory. A similar method, although not sufficient in its own right, is to ask the man to use an alarm to wake himself up at random times during several nights' sleep, preferably during the first few hours when REM sleep occurs most often. Each time he checks if he has an erection. The presence of a full erection on at least one occasion suggests that either there is no physical abnormality or this is having only a small effect. However, an absence of erections on all occasions does not confirm that the cause is physical.

Penile blood pressure can be measured using a paediatric blood pressure cuff and a Dopler ultrasound technique. The ratio of the penile systolic pressure to the systolic pressure measured in the patient's arm can be used to assess for vascular obstruction in the penis (Wagner 1981b).

Corpus cavernosography is a technique in which the pattern of drainage from the penis of a radiological contrast medium is observed. It can be used in the identification of abnormal leakage of blood from the carvernous bodies of the penis, which may cause persistent failure or weakening of erection (Wagner 1981b).

Radiological studies of the pelvic arteries can help identify occlusions which may be causing erectile dysfunction (Michal 1982).

The sensory reflex from the penis to the sacral spinal cord can be tested by measuring evoked nerve potentials in response to applying a tiny electrical stimulus to the skin of the penis. Although this does not directly test the nerves associated with erectile function, it can assist in the evaluation of damage to these nerves or to the spinal cord (Siroky *et al.* 1979).

Finally, measuring with a strain gauge erections evoked by viewing erotic films or slides is another means of evaluating erectile potential (Wagner 1981b).

Women. Apart from a general physical examination, specific examination of the genitalia, and hormone studies, are all that is routinely available for differential diagnosis of sexual disorders in women. A vaginal examination is definitely indicated in all cases of vaginismus and dyspareunia, and in women who have specific anxieties about their genital anatomy. The vagina should be examined for evidence of congenital abnormalities. In women with vaginismus, the vaginal examination will usually replicate the response that occurs when vaginal penetration is attempted by the partner. There may be spasm of the vaginal muscles, tight closing of the thighs, and even arching of the woman's back. The woman can be encouraged to discuss her feelings and anxieties while the examination is carried out. In cases of dyspareunia the vaginal examination can identify an unruptured hymen or tender hymenial remnants, infections, a Bartholin's cyst, postoperational scarring, including a poorly healed episiotomy scar, and thinning of the vaginal wall. Tenderness to deep vaginal examination may result from pelvic inflammatory disease, endometriosis, retroversion of the uterus and ovarian tumours. A vaginal examination should only be carried out by someone with gynaecological experience. Male therapists are reminded *always* to have a female chaperone present while carrying out a vaginal examination.

Hormonal investigations in women are more complicated than in men because of the menstrual cycle. In addition, less is known about hormonal causes of sexual dysfunction in women. When a therapist suspects hormonal abnormality, this should be discussed with or investigated by a gynaecologist.

CONCLUSIONS

Assessment interviews with both partners should always be carried out before a therapist considers offering a couple sex therapy. The main aims of assessment are, first, to find if the couple are suitable for therapy, and secondly, to provide the therapist with a clear picture of the nature of their problem and an understanding of why it developed. In addition, the assessment can itself be therapeutic. Factors which suggest that a couple are unsuitable for sex therapy (and that they may require some other form of treatment) are a very poor general relationship, poor motivation, current severe psychiatric disorder (including alcoholism), untreated physical illness, a current affair by either partner, and pregnancy. This chapter has included details of an assessment schedule. In addition, the indications for and nature of a physical examination, blood tests and other special investigations have been described.

TABLE 6.1

Areas which should be covered during the assessment of each partner

1. The nature and development of the sexual problem
2. Family background and early childhood
3. Early sexual development and experiences, including homosexuality
4. Sexual information
5. Relationship with the partner

   its development
   sexual relationship
   general relationship
   children and contraception
   infidelity
   commitment
6. Schooling and occupation
7. Interests
8. Religious beliefs
9. Medical history
10. Psychiatric history
11. Use of alcohol and drugs (including smoking)
12. Appearance and mood (mental state)
13. Goals and motivation
14. Physical examination and investigations (if necessary)

TABLE 6.2

Aspects of the physical examination and some investigations which may assist in the differential diagnosis of sexual disorders of men

1. *General physical examination*

   General signs of illness: diabetes (e.g. retinopathy), thyroid disorders, adrenal
   cortex disorders
   Hair distribution
   Gynaecomastia
   Blood pressure
   Peripheral pulses (limbs)
   Reflexes (limbs)
   Sensation (limbs)

2. *Genital examination*

   Penis: congenital abnormalities, size, symmetry, tenderness, retractability of
   foreskin, pulses, signs of plaques (Peyronie's disease), infection, urethral discharge
   Testicles: size, symmetry, texture, sensation

3. *Blood tests*

   Testosterone
   LH
   Glucose-fasting (glucose tolerance test if abnormal or diabetes strongly sus-
   pected)
   Prolactin (if testosterone abnormally low)

4. *Special investigations*

     (i) Nocturnal penile tumescence
    (ii) Penile pressure
   (iii) Corpus cavernosography
    (iv) Arteriography of genital blood supply
     (v) Sacral cord evoked potentials
    (vi) Visual stimulation and penile tumescence

7

The formulation

RATIONALE

After a couple have been thoroughly assessed, the next step is for the therapist to discuss with them a formulation of their problem. This has four main purposes:

1. *It should provide the partners with further understanding of their difficulties.* A simple explanation of the nature of the problem and the factors that have contributed to it can assist a couple to see that the problem is not in some way magical or the result of events which cannot be understood. Hence it can provide them with encouragement and enhance the extent of their co-operation with treatment. It can also help them to recognize that there are others with similar problems.

2. *It can encourage a sense of optimism about the outcome of treatment.* During the formulation, the therapist should explain how factors which appear to maintain the problem can be dealt with and how treatment can therefore allow the couple to gain mastery over their difficulties.

3. *It provides a rational basis for the treatment approach.* By explaining how factors such as anxiety can inhibit normal sexual response, and how different causal factors relate to each other, the therapist can demonstrate to a couple why a sex therapy approach to their problem is likely to help them. Thus, for example, a couple are more likely to appreciate the reasons why the therapist suggests a temporary ban on sexual intercourse and asks them initially to begin therapy with non-genital sensate focus (p. 128) if it is explained how a problem associated with sexual

intercourse (e.g. premature ejaculation) can adversely affect the rest of a sexual relationship. Similarly, the therapist can explain how a step-by-step approach will help pin-point more precisely the causes of the couples's problem, and thereby facilitate treatment.

4. *It enables the therapist to check that the information obtained in the assessment has been correctly interpreted.* After presenting the formulation the therapist should ask the couple if it seems to be in keeping with their understanding of their difficulties. Usually a couple will endorse the therapist's account. However, occasionally a couple will reveal new information at this point, or suggest other ways in which the problem may have developed. Thus the formulation can encourage the couple to define and clarify their problems more precisely.

In addition, construction of a formulation can help ensure that the therapist extracts the most relevant points from the information obtained during the assessment. It also demonstrates to a couple that the therapist has both been listening to their accounts and bringing expertise to bear in appraising the information. Finally, it provides a useful initial stage of therapy which can serve as a reference point during subsequent treatment. Thus, in trying to help a couple understand difficulties which they have encountered in treatment, the therapist might refer to the causal factors which were discussed in the formulation.

Content of the formulation

There are two major components to the formulation: first, a description of the problem or problems, and secondly, discussion of the factors which may have caused the problem.

The description of the problem should be brief and simple, but can include a reminder of how it developed. As was discussed in Chapter 6, the therapist should ensure that the partners understand any terms which are used. The couple might be given a name for the problem (e.g. 'vaginismus', 'premature ejaculation').

In describing the causes of the problem the therapist should explain which of them are hypothetical and which are established facts. It is usually helpful if the therapist covers this part of the formulation in terms of the three temporal aspects of causation that were described in Chapter 5. Thus factors in the partners' backgrounds (e.g. inhibited upbringing; being given information which implied sex was something bad) which may have *predisposed* them to developing a sexual problem should be discussed first. Secondly, the therapist should point out any factors which appear to have *precipitated* the problem (e.g. puerperal depression; stress in the couple's general relationship). Finally, the therapist should emphasize the factors which appear to be *maintaining* the problem (e.g. performance anxiety; failure of communication).

As far as possible, the therapist should try to strike a balance between the partners in terms of their individual contributions to the sexual problem. This will help to reduce the likelihood of the partners beginning treatment with the view that only one of them is responsible, although sometimes this is clearly not possible. Nevertheless, the therapist should emphasize that the problem should be regarded as a joint one. Thus, if the problem appears to have originated with one partner, or if one partner brought the problem into the relationship, the couple should be reminded that it affects both of them and that overcoming it requires their equal co-operation and full involvement in therapy. Significant failure of one partner to accept this is often a prelude to a poor outcome.

In the formulation the therapist should emphasize positive aspects of the relationship and each partner's development, as well as indicating negative factors. This might include, for example, reminding them of times when they had satisfactory sexual experiences together, pointing out the enjoyable aspects of their relationship, and noting the extent of their motivation to solve their problem. This is to encourage the couple to feel that their problem is not overwhelming, and that they have sufficient resources to tackle it with reasonable expectation of success.

Above all else, the formulation must be simple and brief. Providing a detailed formulation of the kind that might be presented to a case conference is likely to be unhelpful. Overloading a couple with information, which is very easily done, will only confuse them. A couple may find it helpful if the therapist lists the causal factors on a blackboard while presenting the formulation. If this information is then recorded in the couple's notes the therapist can, if necessary, refer back to it at a later date.

Once the formulation has been presented and discussed, which should only take about 15-20 minutes, the therapist can provide the instructions for the initial homework assignments (Chapter 8).

Example of a formulation

Jane, aged 24, and Peter, aged 31, were referred for sex therapy because of Jane's general lack of interest in sex, and, in particular, her dislike of sexual intercourse. They had been married for 15 months during which time their sexual relationship had never been good, and it had steadily deteriorated until it had ceased altogether.

After a thorough assessment of both partners the couple were offered treatment. During the formulation the therapist explained how as a result of experiences earlier in their lives both partners had become vulnerable to developing sexual difficulties. Thus, Jane came from a family in which sex was never discussed openly. Her mother had given her the impression that sex was dirty. When she unexpectedly had her first period her mother only told her what to do, not what it implied. She had received no proper sex education and her sexual information was limited. Her first sexual experience had been with a much older man; this had caused her to feel guilty and had given her no pleasure. Shortly after she had ended the relationship he had died in a car crash and Jane always wondered whether she had been responsible for this in some way. Peter's sexual development had been straightforward. However, his first wife suddenly left him for another man and this had undermined his self-confidence in his sexual abilities.

Jane and Peter's relationship had developed very rapidly, but when they started to have sex both of them were very hesitant. This precipitated the problem. Jane found it increasingly difficult to become aroused and sexual intercourse was then painful because of inadequate vaginal lubrication. The repeated painful experiences caused her to feel increasingly tense whenever sexual activity began, until eventually she even felt anxious when Peter tried to be affectionate. Not surprisingly, Peter's lack of confidence had steadily increased.

The maintaining factors were (a) Jane and Peter's expectations that each episode of sex would prove an unpleasant failure; (b) their consequent anxiety; and (c) their inability either to discuss the problem or share their anxieties.

The therapist encouraged the couple to feel optimistic about the outcome of treatment by, in particular, pointing out that their general relationship was a happy one and that they both felt very loving towards each other. In addition, they were able to discuss their feelings very openly, provided the topic of sex was avoided, and the problem was not very long-standing.

Summary of the formulation

The summary which was recorded in this couple's notes was as follows:

Predisposing factors:

(1) Jane's inhibited upbringing; encouraged to regard sex as dirty

(2) Her lack of sex education and consequent poor knowledge about sexuality

(3) Guilt about first sexual relationship

(4) Peter's self-confidence undermined by first wife's departure

Precipitants:

(1) Hesitant first sexual experiences together

(2) Jane's sexual arousal impaired—sexual intercourse therefore painful—subsequent anticipatory anxiety

Maintaining factors:

(1) Expectation of failure

(2) Anxiety

(3) Poor communication

CONCLUSIONS

The formulation is an integral part of the sex therapy programme. It provides an excellent basis from which a couple can embark on the homework assignments because it can help them understand their difficulties, encourage them to be optimistic, provide a rationale for the treatment approach, and ensure that the therapist has fully assembled and interpreted the information obtained during the assessment interviews. Often the therapist can only put forward hypothetical reasons for a couple's problem, but can explain how the graduated programme of homework assignments, and the discussions in treatment sessions, should clarify more precisely the reasons for the problem.

8

The homework assignments

The homework assignments for couples constitute the behavioural framework around which sex therapy is conducted. In this chapter the homework assignments are described in detail sufficient for the therapist embarking on sex therapy. In many ways the behavioural programme is quite straightforward. The management of the difficulties which most couples encounter during treatment requires greater skill, and this is considered in detail in the next chapter.

The guidelines in this chapter are derived from those introduced by Masters and Johnson (1970), and developed by Kaplan (1974), but have been supplemented and modified on the basis of subsequent clinical experience.

GENERAL ASPECTS OF THE PROGRAMME

General principles

The behavioural programme has three main purposes:
1. *To provide a structured approach which allows couples to rebuild their sexual relationships gradually.* Thus, it consists of a series of relatively small steps which a couple can tackle one at a time.
2. *To help* a couple and their therapist *identify the specific factors which are maintaining the sexual dysfunction.* The behavioural programme usually highlights features of each partner's

sexuality, and of the interaction between the partners, which are contributing to the sexual problem. The therapist must examine how the partners tackle the homework assignments. This will help to elucidate the attitudes and interactional dynamics of the couple. The therapist must then help the couple relate these to their sexual difficulty in order to further their understanding and thereby assist them to overcome the problem.

3. *To provide a couple with specific techniques to deal with particular problems.* Examples of these are the stop-start or squeeze techniques for overcoming premature ejaculation, and graduated vaginal penetration to reduce penetration fears associated with vaginismus.

First we will consider the basic programme of homework assignments used in the treatment of most couples requiring sex therapy. This includes the stages of:

(1) non-genital sensate focus;
(2) genital sensate focus;
(3) vaginal containment;
(4) vaginal containment with movement.

Then the specific instructions for each type of dysfunction will be described.

In several places the problems which typically occur at the various stages of sex therapy will be discussed, together with some of their causes. Some guidelines to assist in helping couples overcome these difficulties will be provided here. However, because of the great importance of this aspect of therapy, most of the next chapter has been devoted to a more detailed discussion of how to help couples when they encounter difficulties during sex therapy. Sexual problems are often related to general relationship issues, and these usually become apparent during sex therapy. Solution of these difficulties often demands special approaches, and so this aspect of therapy is also considered in a separate chapter (Chapter 11).

The treatment approach described here can be used with most couples. However, the emphasis of therapy should be modified according to the needs, particular problems and progress of each couple. The therapist must be prepared to be flexible; rigidly following a stereotyped programme will result in unnecessary treatment failures.

There are several important principles, listed in Table 8.1, adherence to which should help inexperienced therapists avoid some common mistakes:

1. Always ensure that instructions are clear, and check that the couple have understood them. It is worthwhile repeating instructions, and also asking the couple to repeat them back before the therapy session ends.

2. Before ending a session, find out what the immediate reactions of the partners are to the latest instructions, and whether they anticipate any difficulties. It is often possible to prevent problems by discussing anticipated difficulties.

3. At the beginning of each treatment session, always obtain detailed feedback about a couple's progress since the previous session. It is usually difficult for a therapist to help a couple unless it is clear what they have been doing in their homework sessions, and how they have felt about them.

4. Do not react with disappointment if a couple fail to do or enjoy what was suggested. Difficult patches will occur in the treatment of nearly all couples, and are to be expected. What is more, these are often the times when the reasons for a sexual problem become clearer. Difficulties during the programme, provided these are managed skilfully (Chapter 9), are often crucial in the eventual success of therapy.

5. A most important principle is that *it is unwise to suggest that a couple move on to the next stage in the behavioural programme until the current stage has been mastered.* The pace at which

TABLE 8.1

General guidelines for therapists

1. Give clear instructions and check that they have been understood

2. Ask about anticipated difficulties

3. Obtain detailed feedback

4. View failures or difficulties as offering a chance to increase understanding

5. Adjust the pace of therapy to each couple's progress

6. Avoid introducing uncertainty

7. Make predictions

8. Have regular 'review sessions'

different couples move through the programme will vary according to the nature of their problems and the factors causing them (p. 158).

6. It is inadvisable to leave a couple with the option of moving from one stage in the programme to another, between treatment sessions, even if there is an unusually long delay before the next session. This can lead to uncertainty and hence cause anxiety, especially if the couple are apprehensive about the next stage.

7. Therapists are advised to predict what they think will happen between treatment sessions. Formulation of predictions about how possible causal factors identified in the assessment are likely to affect a couple's responses to the challenge of the homework assignments, and comparison of these with the couple's actual responses, will enable the therapist to develop further understanding of the couple's difficulties.

8. Certain treatment sessions should be designated as 'review sessions'. This policy should be adopted from the outset, the couple being told that their progress will be reviewed after, say, three treatment sessions. Apart from helping to motivate a couple, it can provide a useful 'escape route' for either the therapist or the couple. It should be made clear that if at that stage the therapist, or the partners, should think that the treatment approach is unsuitable they reserve the right to stop. The early review session is suggested because by the third session it is apparent with some couples that the eventual outcome will be poor (p. 206).

Weekly treatment sessions form an efficient and acceptable schedule for most couples and therapists. Although Masters and Johnson's programme includes daily interviews, there is now evidence to suggest that less frequent treatment sessions may be more effective (p. 210). Weekly sessions allow couples more time to practise, and also fit comfortably into the schedules of most therapists. Treatment sessions should not last longer than an hour; they need only last 20-30 minutes when progress is good.

How to introduce the treatment programme

A general introduction, including an overview of the treatment programme, should precede any detailed instructions. The following points should be emphasized:

1. The pace of the programme will be geared to the couple's needs and progress. Some couples or individual partners are fearful that too much will be demanded of them too soon.

2. The couple should approach the programme with a sense of starting afresh, putting previous failures behind them.

3. The couple must make overcoming their sexual problem a major priority in their lives. Distractions should be kept to a minimum. This may mean rearrangements, so that they have fewer visitors and less time is spent in individual pursuits. The partners must ensure that they will have plenty of time together.

4. The couple should expect to encounter difficult patches during therapy. They should not regard failures or difficulties as terrible setbacks, but as providing an opportunity for them, with the help of the therapist, to develop a better understanding of their problems.

5. The major responsibility for mastering the sexual problem lies with the couple. The therapist's role is primarily that of providing a reasonable approach to the problem and helping them learn from mistakes or failures.

6. Some couples, probably because of reading sensational reports in the media, ask if they will have to perform sexual acts in the clinic! It is probably worth explaining to all couples that this is not the case.

7. Discussions during treatment sessions will always be confidential (p. 156).

The couple should then be given some idea of how long treatment will take, how many treatment sessions will occur, and what follow-up arrangements, if any, will be made (see Chapter 12).

Where to begin

Most couples should begin with non-genital sensate focus, the instructions for which are discussed below. However, this is occasionally inappropriate, and the following are three situations in which other strategies would be used at the beginning of treatment.

General disharmony and resentment between the partners may prevent the possibility of their enjoying any physical interaction. The importance of detecting couples for whom general marital rather than sex therapy is indicated has already been discussed (p. 98). In some couples, however, the general difficulties appear to be relatively superficial and can be tackled briefly before a sex therapy programme begins. Specific approaches to general relationship difficulties are discussed in Chapter 11.

Severe phobic aversion in one partner to physical contact remotely associated with sexual activity is another reason for not starting with non-genital sensate focus. For such a couple the phobic partner might be instructed in relaxation exercises to be practised regularly for a week or two. These might then be combined with a programme of imaginal systematic desensitization in which a graduated hierarchy of mild to moderately anxiety-inducing sexual situations are visualized while in a relaxed state (Lazarus 1963; Wincze and Caird 1976). Physical contact with the partner might begin with holding hands, with an explicit ban on any more intimate or extensive physical contact. When such a couple are eventually able to embark on sensate focus, they may have to begin this more or less fully clothed.

Sometimes a couple's problem appears to be very circumscribed, their sexual relationship otherwise being satisfactory. This is occasionally the case, for example, with premature ejaculation. A full sex therapy programme might be unnecessary, as brief counselling may be sufficient (p. 230). However, clinical experience suggests that the early stages of the sex therapy programme can be so beneficial that most couples should be advised to spend at least a week or two practising sensate focus before trying the specific techniques necessary to tackle their particular problem. Furthermore, the relaxed approach to sexuality which results from sensate focus is sometimes sufficient to eliminate the presenting problem.

The general programme of homework assignments used in the treatment of most couples is described below. The strategies for specific problems will be considered later (p. 140).

NON-GENITAL SENSATE FOCUS

Initial instructions

1. The partners are asked to agree, first, not to have sexual intercourse and, secondly, not to touch each other's genitals or

the woman's breasts, until these stages of sexual interaction are reached during the programme. The couple should be informed that this is to ensure that they are not continually confronted by those aspects of sexuality most likely to provoke anxiety, and to allow them to begin to rebuild their sexual relationship by first learning to enjoy general physical contact. This instruction is often received with relief by one or both partners. Occasionally, a couple express the fear that withholding from sexual intercourse will be difficult, impossible, or even damaging for the man or, more rarely, the woman. Using the principle introduced earlier in this chapter, and expounded more fully in the next chapter, the therapist should treat such a response as providing useful information about the couple's attitudes toward sexuality, and should explore this further. For example, this response from the man may reflect performance anxiety (p. 68), whereas such a response by the woman may indicate a basic misunderstanding about sexuality. Another response is that the homework sessions will be so arousing that the couple will not be able to control themselves. The therapist should respond by saying that this stage is not intended to be arousing, but that if sexual arousal occurs the couple should aim to enjoy their feelings without pressurizing each other to have intercourse.

2. During the following week, one partner, when he or she feels like it, should invite the other partner for a homework session. The invitation should be explicit (e.g. 'I feel like trying out those caressing exercises. Do you want to?'), rather than ambiguous, such as turning off the television earlier than usual, or moving closer on the settee. An ambiguous invitation can easily be ignored, whereas unambiguous invitations may improve communication. The other partner should accept the invitation if he or she is either feeling *positive* or *neutral* about having a session. If feeling *negative*, this partner should turn down the invitation, trying, if possible, to explain why.

The aims of these instructions are threefold: first, to encourage both partners to feel confident enough to make themselves vulnerable by asking for what they desire; secondly, to encourage each of the partners to take responsibility for whether or not a session occurs; thirdly, to provide an acceptable means whereby the partners can protect themselves (rather than one partner, for example, always feeling obliged to have sex, should the other wish it); and fourthly, to help the partners improve their communication about sex.

It can usually be left to the couple to determine which partner offers the first invitation. However, if one partner has always felt pressurized because the other partner always instigates sexual activity, the first partner might be asked to provide the initial invitation. Also, if one partner is particularly anxious about the sessions it may be worth suggesting that he or she invites first, in order to alleviate this anxiety as soon as possible

After the first session of caressing, the pattern of inviting then alternates, so that the onus is on the other partner to invite next time.

3. The caressing sessions should occur wherever and whenever the couple wish. They should ensure that they will not be interrupted, and also that they will be warm and comfortable. The eventual aim is that the sessions should occur with both partners naked, and with low lighting. If the couple object to being naked, the therapist should find out why this is so, but should also be flexible. Thus it might be suggested that the partners begin with the least amount of clothing that is acceptable to them. Similarly, a couple might not feel able to begin with the lights on. Again, the therapist should find out why, but also agree to them starting with the lights off, or suggest the use of a very low light placed either behind some furniture or below the level of the bed. The rationale for having lighting should be explained—namely that seeing the partner, and witnessing his or her pleasure, can be very important in a sexual relationship.

Couples often benefit from having the sessions somewhere other than in the setting which has become associated with failure (e.g. the sitting room rather than the bedroom). Some couples also find it pleasant to begin sessions with a mutual bath or shower. They might begin their caressing there.

4. Non-genital sensate focus begins by one partner exploring and caressing the other's body all over, except for the 'no-go areas' (both partners' genitals and the woman's breasts). Kissing, and caressing with the mouth, are included. The partner who gave the invitation for this session starts the caressing. For the purpose of clarity we will suppose that it is the woman who has initiated the session. She should caress her partner in any way that *she herself likes*, but at the same time be aware of how her

partner is enjoying her caresses. The man should focus his attention on the sensations elicited by his partner's caressing. He should let her know what he likes, what he dislikes, and how her caresses could be improved (e.g. by being firmer or lighter, slower or faster). If he finds it difficult to say, he should place his hands on hers and direct her caresses to his liking. While remaining alert to her partner's signals, the woman should try not to guess or worry about what the man is thinking or feeling—if nothing is said she should assume that all is well.

When the partners feel they have had enough of doing things this way round they should tell each other; then the second part of the session begins. The partners swap round and, continuing our example, the man now caresses the woman.

The couple are told to stop should the session become boring or provoke serious anxiety in either partner. Otherwise, the duration of the session, and of each part of it, depends on what feels right for them. Thus a session might last a few minutes, or much longer, such as an hour or more.

5. The main aim of the caressing sessions is for the partners to begin to feel a sense of trust and closeness. In addition, the partners should try to develop greater awareness of what each of them likes and dislikes. The aim of this stage is not that of inducing sexual arousal, although this may happen. The couple are told that if it does, they should try and enjoy the experience of arousal, but avoid going beyond the agreed limits of their caressing.

6. The couple should decide how often they have caressing sessions. However, the therapist should explain that progress will depend to a large extent on how often they have sessions, and that a minimum of three sessions per week would be reasonable.

7. A lotion applied sparingly to the skin is generally a pleasant adjunct to the caressing. This is not usually suggested until after a week or so of sensate focus. It is most important to avoid any lotion likely to have irritant properties (especially if it is to be used later on the genitals). Baby-lotion (warmed if necessary) is very useful for this purpose (K-Y jelly is another possibility). Some couples prefer to use talcum powder rather than a lotion.

8. There is no restriction on masturbation, should either partner wish to relieve sexual tension, but for the present this should be restricted to self-masturbation, not in the partner's presence.

9. The homework sessions might be found artificial or contrived.

However, with persistence, most couples find them very enjoyable.

10. The partners should try to use the personal pronoun 'I' as much as possible, not just during sensate focus (e.g. 'I need to know how you are feeling about what I am doing', rather than 'You don't seem to be enjoying this') but also in their day-to-day interactions with each other. This encourages them to take responsibility for personal statements and avoids ambiguous communication (e.g. 'I do not want to go out this evening' rather than 'Why do we have to go out this evening?').

After giving the initial instructions concerning sensate focus, and checking that the partners have fully understood them, the therapist should prepare the couple for the next treatment session, explaining that they will need to review in detail how they have progressed during the first week. This will make it easier for the therapist to ask detailed questions at the next session, which can otherwise be difficult because of fear of causing embarrassment. As was noted earlier, the therapist should make private predictions concerning what will happen, basing these on the information obtained in the initial assessment interviews and the couple's reactions to the initial instructions.

The second treatment session

A good opening to the second interview is to ask both partners to say in general how they have progressed since the previous session. The therapist should then proceed to obtain from each partner a detailed account of what occurred, and their reaction to the sessions, including both positive and negative experiences. It is important to avoid simply accepting statements such as 'It was fine' or 'It didn't work'; the therapist must gain a full understanding of what occurred. This is necessary not only to ensure that the therapist has sufficient information, but also because detailed discussion of the homework sessions can encourage the partners to communicate more easily with each other about their sexual relationship.

Reactions to non-genital sensate focus

The initial reactions of a couple to non-genital sensate focus may be positive, negative, or, and perhaps more commonly, a mixture of the two.

For some couples these exercises provide a profoundly positive experience, in which they are able to enjoy relaxed physical inter-action for the first time ever, or at least for a very long time. This may result in a change in the way the partners behave towards each other, which is obvious in the treatment sessions in which they may appear closer and more affectionate than previously. Often, however, the initial reactions are negative, or the couple have not kept within the agreed limits. Couples commonly report back in the following ways:

(1) the sessions lacked spontaneity, and seemed artificial and contrived;

(2) there was not enough time to have any sessions, or to have more than one session;

(3) the ban was broken, with the couple going on to have sexual intercourse;

(4) the sessions evoked negative feelings, such as tension in one or both partners, ticklishness, boredom ('mind wandering'), or finding the partner clumsy;

(5) one partner could not bring himself or herself to offer an invitation.

The ways in which the therapist should deal with these and other similar responses are discussed in detail in the next chapter. The important thing is to try first to help the couple understand their responses. For example, the therapist might relate their difficulties to possible causal factors identified during the assessment interviews. Only then should further suggestions be offered, or the partners asked for suggestions as to how they might be able to get the most out of their sessions.

The therapist should not advise a couple to proceed to the next stage of the programme until they have been able to enjoy several sessions of non-genital sensate focus, otherwise the considerable benefits of this stage will be missed and any difficulties are likely to be compounded later. Sometimes, in order to provide a more gradual progression to the next stage, and to maintain a couple's sense of progress, the therapist might suggest that the caressing sessions are extended to include the woman's breasts.

GENITAL SENSATE FOCUS

Instructions
In this next phase of the programme the partners should continue

their pattern of alternate inviting. Initially, they should also continue to begin each session with one partner active and the other passive, swapping these roles midway through the session. Now it is suggested that they include the woman's breasts and both partner's genitals in their caressing. It is important, especially when there is anxiety about this stage, to instruct each partner to extend caressing in this way only when the other partner is prepared for it.

During the first few sessions of genital sensate focus the caressing should be gentle and exploratory. The partners should not strive to become aroused, nor put pressure on each other to do so. Instead, they should concentrate on the relaxed giving and receiving of erotic pleasure. The couple should try to relax and enjoy the feelings of arousal. Later during this stage the couple should concentrate more on arousing each other. In addition, they can try to allow their sexual arousal to wax and wane.

The therapist must describe the exercises in some detail. For example, the man should lightly stroke around the entrance to the woman's vagina. He should be discouraged initially from putting his fingers right inside the vagina, because his partner may not find this pleasurable (p. 9); for some women, especially those suffering from vaginismus, this is likely to cause acute anxiety. The man should also lightly touch his partner's clitoris, but only when she is becoming aroused, otherwise this might be uncomfortable. He should concentrate not just on the genital area, but also caress his partner's thighs and lower abdomen, as well as her breasts. His attention should switch from one part of the body to another. The woman should let her partner know how she is feeling, either verbally or by showing her feelings in some other way such as by nodding or smiling. The hand-on-hand means of guiding the partner (p. 131) can be very useful during this stage. The couple should use whatever position they wish, but many couples find what Masters and Johnson (1970) described as the 'non-demand position' particularly helpful when the man is doing the caressing: the man sits with his back comfortably supported by pillows, and the woman sits between his legs with her back against his chest and her head resting on his shoulder. The woman may feel secure in this position, and it allows her partner to caress her breasts and genitals. A man who has erectile dysfunction will often begin to experience erections again in this position. While caressing her partner the woman should also caress his thighs and lower abdomen. Stroking of his penis should initially be gentle; she should also caress his scrotum. Her attention should move from his genitals to other parts of his body, and then return to the genitals. Some men find it difficult to lie back and passively receive erotic pleasuring of this kind. They may experience anxiety resulting from activation of performance needs. The therapist might anticipate this potential difficulty, emphasizing that developing the ability to become aroused in this way will greatly add to the man's pleasure. It is essential that men with premature ejaculation learn to do this before the stop-start or squeeze techniques (p. 149) are suggested.

The couple are told that they can use their hands or lips in their caressing as they wish. The topic of oral sex should be raised at this stage. Oral sex should not be a mandatory part of the programme, but couples should be allowed to make up their own minds about whether they include oral sex in their sexual repertoires. However, it is often a source of disagreement, usually because one partner likes the idea and the other does not, and the therapist should then help the partners discuss the issue, and assist them to resolve it. The therapist must explain that there are no fixed rules, but that some people find oral sex an intensely pleasurable part of sexuality, whereas others feel no need for it. Some couples can reach a compromise so that oral stimulation is only provided by one partner.

Couples who have been using a lotion during non-genital sensate focus should be encouraged to continue using it during genital caressing. It will often add to their pleasure, and will be particularly useful in the later stages of treatment of both vaginismus (p. 144) and retarded ejaculation (p. 151). When treating premature ejaculation, however, the therapist should suggest that the lotion is not used initially during genital caressing of the man because he may find that his ejaculatory response is accelerated.

Both partners should now concentrate on caressing in a way that gives pleasure to the other partner, as well as to themselves. Each must, therefore, carefully attend to feedback from the other. Both partners should try to 'stay with' pleasurable feelings, and avoid being distracted. At the end of a session they may, if they wish, go on to experience orgasm. However, initially this should not be a goal of the sessions.

Once the genital sensate focus exercises have been successfully incorporated into the couple's homework sessions, with the partners alternating between the active and passive roles, the couple are then advised to caress each other simultaneously while retaining the alternating pattern for part of the session. However, they should continue their pattern of alternately initiating sessions.

Specific techniques for dealing with particular sexual difficulties will be introduced at this stage. These are discussed later in this chapter (p. 140).

Reactions to genital sensate focus

Some couples are immediately able to enjoy genital sensate focus in a relaxed fashion, with rapid and intense arousal. This may in some cases lead to breaking the ban on sexual intercourse, but this should be discouraged.

Negative reactions are very common, even though a couple may have enjoyed several successful sessions of non-genital sensate focus. This stage is particularly likely to generate sexual anxiety. This may be mild, and disappear after a few sessions of pleasuring. In other cases it is severe, and results either in avoidance and eventual cessation of homework sessions, or in the sessions becoming increasingly unpleasant for one or both partners.

The presentation and management of such negative reactions are discussed fully in the next chapter. However, the main points will be summarized here. Difficulties at this stage may become apparent because, for example, a couple report:

(1) breaking the agreed ban on sexual intercourse. Although, as noted above, this may reflect a healthy response to erotic pleasure, it may also reflect difficulties, such as performance anxieties, or a need to terminate genital pleasuring because it is unpleasant. Clarifying the extent to which the partners have been able to relax and enjoy genital sensate focus will help differentiate between these two responses;

(2) negative feelings, such as anxiety, ticklishness, numbness,

or even pain. These may lead to avoidance of sessions.

The management of such responses includes:
(1) simply suggesting that the couple repeat the homework assignment; this is appropriate when the negative response is mild;
(2) using the approaches described in the next chapter for identifying negative attitudes and thoughts, if these are not immediately apparent.

Common factors likely to lead to negative responses include general inhibitions, guilt, anxiety about the appearance of the genitals or about sexual odours or secretions, and fear of loss of control by either partner.

(3) suggesting the use of erotic fantasies in order to prevent distraction, and to enhance arousal (pp. 140; 219).

(4) by-passing the part of the programme that is causing anxiety, if it does not seem an essential component in tackling the problem of the particular couple.

VAGINAL CONTAINMENT

Once genital sensate focus is well established, the next step in the programme is the gradual introduction of sexual intercourse via an intermediate stage called *vaginal containment*. One aim of this stage is to minimize the anxiety that is induced in some couples by sexual intercourse. This is common in men who suffer from either premature ejaculation or erectile dysfunction, because sexual intercourse has become associated with failure. Similarly, the idea of vaginal penetration is the main source of anxiety for most women who suffer from vaginismus.

Instructions

The couple should move on to this stage during a session of pleasuring when they are both feeling relaxed and sexually aroused. There are several positions which are suitable for vaginal containment. The male superior, or 'missionary' position, is not usually recommended, for several reasons. For example, it can reduce ejaculatory control in a man with premature ejaculation (perhaps because of increased muscle tone and spinal cord neural activity resulting from the man needing to support his body weight). A woman with vaginismus may particularly dislike this position because she does not feel in control of vaginal penetration.

Either the female-superior position, or the side-by-side or lateral position, are usually suggested. Whatever position is chosen, the therapist should describe it in detail, preferably using an illustration (Kaplan 1974 and 1976 are useful sources). For the female-superior position the woman should sit astride her partner, resting on her knees, ensuring that they are approximately level with his nipples. If she is positioned further down his body, the angle of alignment of her vagina and his penis will be awkward and may cause discomfort for either partner, or prevent penetration altogether. For the lateral position the partners lie side-by-side, facing each other. The woman draws up her knees and the man lies between her legs. Penile penetration in either position should be accomplished by the woman guiding her partner's penis into her vagina with her hands. If the man conducts penetration, fumbling or difficulty finding the vaginal entrance can make the procedure awkward and cause loss of arousal for either or both partners. In a couple with vaginismus, it is also essential for the woman to feel that she has control over vaginal penetration.

Once penetration has occurred, the couple should remain still, concentrating on any pleasant sensations they experience. The man may move a little to stimulate himself if his erection begins to subside. If the woman is able to contract her vaginal muscles (p. 218) she might do this occasionally to enhance both her own and her partner's pleasure. Containment should last however long the partners wish; it might be a few seconds or several minutes, following which they should withdraw and continue their pleasuring. Vaginal containment should be repeated two or three times in any one session. The duration of vaginal containment might gradually be increased on each occasion.

If the couple have been experiencing orgasm during genital sensate focus, they should initially avoid this during containment, but continue to reach orgasm extravaginally. In this way, vaginal containment becomes incorporated in the overall pattern of pleasuring, rather than signalling the termination of sexual activity.

Reactions to vaginal containment

If a couple have been able to enjoy genital sensate focus, and the presenting problem is not specifically concerned with vaginal penetration, vaginal containment is usually accomplished without any difficulty. However, it is not unusual for erectile failure to recur at this stage because of re-awakened anxieties about the need to maintain erection once vaginal penetration has occurred. If a man has been getting and maintaining good erections during genital sensate focus, and has practised the waxing and waning exercise (p. 148), this is usually a temporary problem. Vaginal penetration often causes anxiety, and therefore difficulty, for men with premature ejaculation. Although this may also be temporary, it sometimes indicates that the specific procedure for managing premature ejaculation (p. 148) has not yet been sufficiently well established. Vaginal penetration is of course a crucial stage for women with vaginismus, and specific means of helping them achieve this successfully are described later (p. 142).

VAGINAL CONTAINMENT WITH MOVEMENT

In this stage the couple introduce movement during vaginal containment and gradually progress to full sexual intercourse. It usually represents the final phase of the behavioural programme. It is generally suggested that the woman moves first, doing so in a way that provides her with pleasurable sensations. Later, the man begins to move. Then they might take turns at moving. The movement should at first be slow; only after several sessions should the couple introduce more vigorous movements and re-establish (or establish for the first time) full sexual intercourse.

If a couple have managed vaginal containment successfully this stage does not usually cause any particular problems, except sometimes in the case of premature ejaculation (p. 150).

Finally, the therapist should suggest that the couple try, if they wish, experimenting with different positions for sexual intercourse. These should be described, preferably with the aid of pictures or diagrams. Depending on the nature of the presenting problem, those positions especially suited to providing the woman with clitoral stimulation (female-superior), or to allowing shallow vaginal penetration (rear-entry) might be indicated. The therapist might also suggest that the man uses his fingers to provide his partner with clitoral stimulation during vaginal containment or sexual intercourse.

This completes the general programme of homework assignments. Below are described the techniques which can be used in the management of the specific sexual dysfunctions. These are grafted onto this general programme, according to the nature of a couple's problem.

TECHNIQUES FOR SPECIFIC TYPES OF SEXUAL DYSFUNCTION

The specific types of dysfunction, and the therapeutic techniques that can help overcome them, will be considered in the order used in the classification of sexual dysfunctions in Chapter 3.

Impaired sexual interest

There are no additional specific techniques for this dysfunction, although some of the procedures used for other problems (e.g. Kegel exercises, sexual fantasies, waxing and waning of erections) might be suggested. Therapy is mainly focused on helping the couple resolve general relationship issues (Chapter 11), and on their using the sensate focus programme as a means of gradually re-establishing a satisfactory sexual relationship. Difficulties such as inhibitions about sexual behaviour, fear of sexual arousal, and too limited foreplay, often become apparent during the treatment of this problem.

Impaired sexual arousal

As was noted earlier (p. 33), this is a relatively uncommon problem in pre-menopausal women in the absence of impaired sexual interest. One possible means of increasing arousal is through the use of sexual fantasies. However, because this is a topic which will be regarded with horror by some couples, it must be broached with extreme care. The therapist might reassure a couple that once sexual arousal can occur with fantasies, the need to use them may gradually diminish because arousal will have become associated with their own sexual relationship.

Post-menopausal women who, because of atrophic vaginitis, suffer from impaired vaginal arousal in response to sexual activity, often benefit from using oestrogen cream which is applied to the vaginal wall. This treatment should be supervised by a doctor (usually a gynaecologist) who has experience of its indications and limitations.

Orgasmic dysfunction

The types of homework assignments which might be recommended during the treatment of orgasmic dysfunction will depend on the nature of the presenting problem. If the problem is one of primary total orgasmic dysfunction (i.e. the woman has never experienced a self- or partner-induced orgasm), a masturbation-training programme to be used by the woman alone may be most relevant. This is described in Chapter 14. The programme of sensate focus exercises can continue in parallel with this. However, some couples find this approach unacceptable, and wish to resolve the problem with the man providing all the sexual stimulation that his partner receives, rather than her pleasuring herself.

If the masturbation training programme is used, then once the woman is able to experience orgasm on her own, the next stage is the same as for the woman presenting with situational orgasmic dysfunction (i.e. she cannot experience orgasm with her partner). During genital sensate focus the woman can either demonstrate to her partner how she stimulates herself, or guide his hand to show him how she likes being caressed (e.g. she might place her fingers over her partner's while he massages her clitoris). A teasing approach, in which clitoral stimulation is interspersed with general caressing, often increases sexual excitement. In view of the recent suggestions concerning the sensitivity of the anterior wall of the vagina (p. 10) it might be worth suggesting that the couple explore this in their sessions. If the orgasmic dysfunction persists, use of a vibrator might be suggested (p. 219), although any worries a couple might have about this suggestion must be explored. A common source of concern is the feeling that the use of a sexual aid underlines the couple's sexual inadequacy. Discussion of the range of orgasmic responsivity in women (p. 14), and the fact that the vibrator is only a temporary measure, may help allay this concern.

Once orgasm occurs regularly during genital sensate focus, a bridge manoeuvre (Kaplan 1976) may be used to help the woman experience orgasm during sexual intercourse. This involves the woman receiving clitoral stimulation during vaginal containment, possibly combined with slow pelvic thrusting. The stimulation can be provided by the woman herself, or by her partner. A vibrator might also be used. When the woman feels herself approaching orgasm she should begin vigorous pelvic thrusting, continuing to obtain clitoral stimulation, if possible, by pressing her clitoris against her partner's pelvic bone. This may lead to coital orgasm. However, occasionally, it causes some loss of arousal, in which case the procedure should be repeated. The advantage of having the woman stimulate herself is that she can tune in precisely to her level of arousal and provide the type of stimulation she requires. If the man feels an overwhelming need to ejaculate, he should do so, and then either go back to caressing his partner, or delay using the procedure again until the next session.

Some women will eventually be able to experience orgasm with sexual intercourse alone. However, for perhaps the majority, clitoral stimulation will usually be necessary. Those couples in which the woman cannot eventually experience orgasm during sexual intercourse should be helped to accept that non-coital orgasm is not second-best, and that the woman's experience is similar to that of many other perfectly normal women.

Common reactions to these homework assignments include the woman expressing anger, or feelings of inadequacy, because she views herself as inferior to other women who are able to experience orgasm during sexual intercourse, and a sense of inadequacy on the part of the man who feels he ought to be able to bring his partner to orgasm without resorting to special techniques. In both cases the therapist can often help by explaining the range of orgasmic response found in women (p. 14).

Vaginismus

The approach used with vaginismus consists of helping the woman become more comfortable with her genitals, and gradual exposure to different types of vaginal penetration in order to overcome her fears of penetration. Although the outcome of treatment for vaginismus is generally good, treatment is often not straightforward. Resistance may be encountered at each stage, especially early on, although in nearly every case this can be overcome by encouragement and counselling. Vaginismus can sometimes be overcome solely by means of homework exercises. In other cases the early tasks in the programme must be carried out in the clinic before a couple will feel confident enough to try them at home. Which approach will work usually becomes clear after the couple have tried doing things at home during the first two or three weeks of therapy.

First, most women with vaginismus must become familiar and comfortable with their genitals. As was noted in Chapter 3, some women with vaginismus regard their genitals with distaste, and may have distorted ideas about the size of the vagina, thinking it is far too small ever to accommodate a penis. The woman should begin by examining her genitals with a hand mirror and should repeat this on several occasions. She should identify the various parts of her genital anatomy, which the therapist should already have described using a photograph or diagram (Fig. 2.1). Some women prefer to do this on their own, while others would rather have their partner present.

At this stage the woman is taught the Kegel exercises in order to gain more control over her vaginal muscles. These are described on p. 218.

Next, the woman should gently introduce the tip of one finger into her vaginal entrance. She can do the Kegel exercises at the same time and feel her vaginal muscles tightening and relaxing. Subsequently, she should gradually insert her entire finger into her vagina and explore the inside. When she has been able to do this several times, while remaining relaxed, she should try inserting two fingers, and when feeling confident, gently move them around.

Sometimes a woman is unable to begin this programme unaided, in which case the therapist must intervene more actively. The woman can be taken into a clinical examination room and encouraged to examine herself with a hand mirror, and then to insert a finger into her vagina. If the latter seems too difficult for her, the therapist should carry out a gentle vaginal examination, while assisting the woman to relax by suggesting deep breathing. The woman should be encouraged at the same time to talk about her anxieties concerning vaginal penetration. Although the therapist should use a surgical glove for this examination, the woman should be asked to do it without one. This helps both to preserve an appropriate therapist-patient relationship, and to encourage the woman to accept that her genitals are clean. Male therapists must always have a female chaperone present. These clinic sessions may take place over several weeks, or, if the problem is not a severe one, can be compressed into one. The woman is asked to repeat at home whatever she has been able to do in the treatment session.

In the next stage of treatment the woman's partner repeats what the woman has done, in the context of their pleasuring sessions. First, he should examine her genitals, and then, under her guidance, gently insert into her vagina first a finger tip, and then a whole finger. Subsequently, if possible, he should then insert two fingers. Once the woman can relax during finger penetration, her partner should gently move his finger(s). Again, the number of treatment sessions necessary before this can be accomplished will vary greatly from couple to couple.

Next, the couple are instructed in vaginal containment. The female-superior or lateral positions are best because the woman can retain a sense of control. The couple should use a lubricant (e.g. baby lotion or K-Y jelly) to facilitate penetration. As noted earlier, it is most important that the woman inserts the penis herself. Sometimes, carrying out the Kegel exercises at this point can assist penetration, the penis being inserted as the pubo-coccygeous muscles relax following a contraction. Finally, movement is introduced by the woman during vaginal containment, until eventually the couple are able to have full sexual intercourse.

Many therapists, including Masters and Johnson (1970), use graded vaginal dilators in the treatment of vaginismus. The woman first inserts the smallest dilator into her vagina. When she can do this comfortably, she progresses to using the next biggest, and so on. When she is able to use one of the largest dilators, she shows her partner how to insert them, again beginning with the smallest. Clinical experience has suggested that dilators are not necessary in the treatment of most women with vaginismus, although they might be of use if a woman has great difficulty in transferring from finger to penile penetration.

Treatment of vaginismus often proceeds more rapidly if, as described above, the therapist has the woman practise the early stages in the clinic before trying them at home. However, an entirely home-based approach can be used, especially by non-medical therapists who should not perform vaginal examinations. Should this be unsuccessful, a medically qualified therapist may have to be involved.

Dyspareunia

When dyspareunia is the result of psychological factors causing impaired sexual arousal (and hence painful vaginal penetration and, possibly, deep vaginal pain because of buffeting of the cervix during sexual intercourse (p. 35)), the main goal of therapy is to help the woman to begin to enjoy sexual contact and become sexually aroused. Thus the programme of sensate focus exercises, and exploring the difficulties that it highlights, will be the mainstay of treatment. However, advice on positions for sexual intercourse in which there is unlikely to be full vaginal penetration (see below) may also help by allaying the anxieties of the woman who has become fearful of deep penetration, thus allowing her to relax and enjoy sexual intercourse.

When deep dyspareunia is the result of physical pathology (e.g. pelvic adhesions, endometriosis) which cannot be fully resolved by medical or surgical procedures, advice on positions in which vaginal penetration during sexual intercourse is limited can again be helpful. Rear-entry (side-by-side) or lateral positions are two examples. Some women prefer the female-superior position, in which they can easily control the depth of vaginal penetration.

If a woman reports general vaginal soreness after sexual intercourse, and there is no evidence of vaginal infection or other vaginal pathology, the therapist should be alert to the possibility, albeit rare, that the woman is allergic to her partner's semen. Skin sensitivity tests may help confirm the diagnosis. Use of a condom during sexual intercourse should eliminate the problem.

Sexual phobias

As noted in Chapter 3, sexual phobias usually accompany other more general sexual dysfunctions, such as impaired sexual interest or erectile dysfunction, and the main focus of treatment should therefore be the resolution of the general problem. However, there are specific techniques which can be used in the management of sexual phobias, irrespective of whether the phobia is a distinct problem or part of a broader dysfunction.

The most useful approach is based on graded exposure, in which the problem is broken down into a series of steps of increasing difficulty. The couple are instructed to concentrate on incorporating the first step into their homework sessions until phobic anxiety is eliminated, then to practise the next step, and so on. If necessary, this could be preceded by the imaginal approach described earlier (p. 128).

Graded exposure is illustrated by a woman who had a phobia about her breasts being caressed. She refused to allow her partner to caress her breasts because this made her tense, and sometimes was even painful. The therapist first established that this was not simply the result of clumsy caressing by her partner. Because the problem was clearly of a phobic kind (related to the woman's longstanding embarrassment about early breast development which had led to ridicule by friends), the therapist suggested that during the sensate focus exercises the man should at some stage (determined by the woman) briefly lay a hand on the side of one of her breasts, and then move his hand away to continue caressing elsewhere. The woman said she would feel safer if, initially, she covered her partner's hand with hers. Once this was accomplished without anxiety, the man then left his hand on the breast for longer periods, still without moving. The next step was for the man to provide gentle caressing to the side of the woman's breast. Only when this was established did he then lay his hands on his partner's nipples, again initially without movement. Eventually the woman was able to allow him gently to manipulate and kiss her nipples, and began to experience pleasure from this.

The approach to sexual phobias must not be entirely mechanistic. Success is more likely if the partners have first been able to develop some understanding of the basis of the problem. One illustration of the origins of phobic avoidance of breast stimulation was given above; further reasons for such a phobia might include those of a woman feeling that her breasts are unattractive, too small, too large, etc. These attitudes should be explored further, with the therapist encouraging the man to make his attitudes (which may be very different) known to his partner. Sexual phobias are sometimes based on false beliefs, which the therapist should counteract. One example was a woman who showed phobic avoidance of seminal fluid, which was based on her belief that semen was unhygienic. Once the anxiety had been reduced by providing information, graded exposure was then used to tackle the avoidance. This included suggesting that the woman allow a small drop of semen to remain briefly on her skin, and that she then left it on for increasingly longer periods.

Erectile dysfunction

In most cases of psychogenic erectile dysfunction the man will begin to have erections during either non-genital or genital sensate focus. A useful strategy is to suggest that the man tries *not* to have an erection during the initial stages of the sex therapy programme. Apart from removing the pressure on him to get an erection, this suggestion sometimes appears to enhance the chances that he *will* have an erection. This is an example of a strategy called 'paradoxical intention', which is discussed later (p. 170).

The couple should be encouraged to use a lotion during genital caressing, and the man should try to concentrate entirely on the erotic sensations he is experiencing. Men with erectile difficulties very often focus their attention on whether or not they have an erection and, if they have one, how firm it is. Some couples report greater success when they have their sessions of pleasuring in the mornings soon after waking, when the man's erectile response may be maximal. This can be a very useful suggestion for older couples and in cases where partial erectile dysfunction is the result of a physical disorder, such as diabetes or multiple sclerosis.

If a couple have spent two or three weeks practising genital sensate focus without erections beginning to occur, or with only weak erections, further suggestions can be made. If acceptable to the couple, the man might use sexual fantasies to heighten his erotic pleasure and to prevent distracting negative thoughts. A teasing approach to genital stimulation, in which the woman briefly stimulates her partner's penis, and then moves her attention elsewhere, especially to his scrotum and inner thighs, can be very effective. Oral stimulation, again if acceptable, might also be encouraged.

Once genital sensate focus is well established and the man is having erections, the *waxing and waning* technique should be suggested. During a homework session, once the man has a strong erection, the partners should cease their caressing (genital or non-genital) for a few minutes and allow the erection to subside. They should then resume caressing, with the woman slowly stroking her partner's penis. The man will usually find his erection returns. The procedure can be repeated two or three times in a session. This is an effective means of dispelling the fear that most men with erectile difficulties experience when beginning to lose an erection; at this point they usually become anxious, which results in further loss of erection, and then automatically assume that the erection will not be regained. The waxing and waning procedure can also assist in removing the pressure a man might feel to sustain his erection throughout love play.

Because some couples feel that ejaculation should only occur inside the vagina, and this puts further pressure on the man to maintain an erection once sexual intercourse begins, the man should be encouraged to ejaculate extravaginally. As noted earlier, the moment of penetration often provokes much anxiety for a man with erectile difficulties, because this is the point at which he feels the greatest pressure to keep his erection. The stage of containment is therefore extremely important. The woman should take the responsibility for inserting his penis, because any fumbling on the part of the man may quickly cause his erection to subside. Once his penis is inside the vagina, he can gently thrust in order to provide himself with stimulation, or she can do this. Containment should initially only be brief; the woman might use it as a further extension of her teasing stimulation of her partner. It is not unusual for there to be a few failures at this stage before containment is successful. The therapist should explain that this is to be expected, and encourage the couple to keep practising. Once containment has been successfully accomplished several times, the couple can then proceed through the rest of the programme as described earlier.

Premature ejaculation

The special techniques now available for the treatment of premature ejaculation have made this problem relatively easy to manage in many cases. When at the stage of genital sensate focus, the couple should be instructed in either the 'stop-start' or 'squeeze' techniques. For either of these the man must be able to identify, during his sexual arousal, the point of inevitability after which ejaculation is bound to occur (p. 20). Some men with premature ejaculation are not aware of this point because their sexual response cycle is so rapid. The best way to learn to identify it is during self-masturbation, in which the man tries to prolong arousal while concentrating on erotic sensations.

The *stop-start technique* was first introduced by Semans (1956). In order to practise this the man should lie on his back, focusing his attention fully on the sensations provided by his partner stimulating his penis. His partner can sit alongside him, or between his legs. She should slowly stroke his penis until he indicates that he feels himself become highly aroused, at which point she stops her stroking and allows his arousal to subside. The means by which he communicates high arousal should have been agreed beforehand. He should not wait until he has reached the point of inevitability. After a short delay of no more than a couple of minutes, his partner resumes her stroking and the procedure is repeated. The couple should aim to do this three times, and then, on the fourth occasion, the woman continues stroking until the man ejaculates. The couple should practice this procedure during each session of genital sensate focus. Use of a lotion during genital caressing should be avoided at first, but may be introduced once control has been established. This will add to the man's genital sensations, and will also make genital stimulation more like vaginal containment.

The *squeeze technique*, which was introduced by Masters and Johnson (1970), is probably not necessary unless control does not develop after several attempts with the stop-start approach. In this procedure, when the man indicates high arousal, the woman applies a firm squeeze to the head of his penis for 15-20 seconds. Her forefinger and middle finger are placed over the base of the glans penis and the shaft of the penis, on the upper surface of the penis, and her thumb is placed across the coronal sulcus at the base of the undersurface of the glans penis (Fig. 8.1). The effect of this is to inhibit the ejaculatory reflex. Sometimes there is also partial loss of erection. As with the stop-start technique, this procedure is repeated three times and on the fourth occasion the

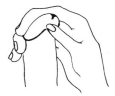

Fig. 8.1 Squeeze technique

man proceeds to ejaculation. Before practising the squeeze technique with the man highly aroused, the woman should apply the squeeze a few times when her partner has an erection in order to find out how firmly she can squeeze without causing pain. This is usually a lot firmer than most couples expect.

With either the stop-start or squeeze techniques the couple should be warned that it is common for there to be a few initial failures, but that persistence usually brings success.

Once extravaginal ejaculatory control is well-established the couple should move on to vaginal containment. The female superior position usually allows a man to have great control over ejaculation (p. 137). As noted earlier, penetration often causes considerable apprehension for men with premature ejaculation, because it has been associated with failure in the past. Setbacks are again to be expected. The man should signal high arousal, as before, and the woman should then lift herself off her partner until his arousal subsides. The couple should use the squeeze technique if this has been in their programme. Movement is gradually introduced, first by the woman, and later by the man. If possible, ejaculation should continue to occur extravaginally at first. Eventually the couple should be able to have full sexual intercourse, using the stop-start as necessary, with or without the man withdrawing his penis from the vagina.

The reaction of some couples to techniques used for premature ejaculation is one of boredom. If this occurs, the therapist must ensure that they are continuing to enjoy their sensate focus exercises. Another reaction is sexual frustration on the part of the woman, in which case the therapist should find out whether the partner is paying enough attention to her pleasure and stimulating her to orgasm if she wishes for this. However, because the man is likely to find his partner's orgasm highly arousing, the couple should practise the control procedure for premature ejaculation first.

Couples often need to continue practising the special techniques for premature ejaculation for several weeks or months before satisfactory control is established during sexual intercourse. They should be told to expect occasional periods in future when ejaculatory control will be reduced. They should then re-introduce the stop-start or squeeze technique until control is regained.

Retarded ejaculation

If, as is usually the case, ejaculatory retardation or failure is situational (i.e. the man can ejaculate when masturbating on his own), during genital sensate focus the man's partner should concentrate first on gentle stimulation of his penis. The couple should use a lotion or K-Y jelly which will increase the man's arousal, and also act as a lubricant. The man should lie on his back and focus his attention on the sensations he is experiencing. Over the space of several sessions the woman should gradually increase the vigour of her stimulation, and also alternate this with more gentle and teasing caressing. If ejaculation occurs, then in the next few sessions the man should ejaculate close to the vaginal entrance. Subsequently, when about to ejaculate, the man should insert his penis into his partner's vagina and continue vigorous thrusting until he ejaculates. If his arousal subsides before ejaculation the procedure should be repeated. In treating retarded ejaculation the male-superior position *is* recommended because this often facilitates ejaculation. Increased stimulation of the glans penis may occur during sexual intercourse if the woman gently pulls the skin at the base of the penis downwards.

Sometimes, a woman will initially be unable to bring her partner to ejaculation by manual stimulation. In this case the man should masturbate in her presence. When he is able to ejaculate, in subsequent sessions the woman should take over stroking of his penis progressively earlier during masturbation until she can bring him to ejaculation herself. Then the programme can proceed as above.

If success is not obtained with these techniques, the couple might try using a vibrator, although most men do not seem to respond as well to vibrators as do women.

For men who have never ejaculated when awake, treatment is best begun with an individual masturbation training programme. This is described later (p. 222). Retarded ejaculation is often difficult to treat. Some men report, for example, that their partner's stroking is not pleasurable. This may be linked to an obsessive need for control. It may occasionally be overcome if the man can begin to use his most arousing fantasies. Such a response sometimes reflects a powerful wish to avoid abandonment with the partner because of feelings of hostility. Usually this can only be identified by careful exploration as described in the next chapter.

Sexual phobias

The behavioural approaches to sexual phobias in men are similar to those described for women with such problems (p. 145). Sometimes a man's phobia about sexual activity is the result of him disliking his partner's abandonment when she is very aroused. This difficulty may arise out of double-standards about female sexuality, exploration of which is discussed later (p. 165).

CONCLUSIONS

The homework assignments described in this chapter form the behavioural framework of sex therapy. The general programme, which begins with sensate focus, can be used with most couples. Other strategies will depend on the nature of a couple's sexual difficulties. The therapist must plan out a programme to meet each couple's needs. The pace at which this proceeds will depend on the couple's progress and the problems they encounter. For most couples, advice on the homework assignments alone will be insufficient, and difficulties are nearly always encountered during treatment. Sometimes these can be overcome by simple modification of the programme, or through sex education as described in Chapter 10. In many cases, however, the therapist must help a couple understand what is causing the difficulty and find ways round it. Most of the next chapter is devoted to this aspect of treatment.

9

Maximizing therapeutic effects and overcoming difficulties

The general nature of the interactions between therapist and couple during sex therapy is an important factor in determining eventual outcome. This relationship is therefore considered in some detail in the first part of this chapter.

The programme of homework assignments in sex therapy has a dual purpose. The first is to provide the couple with an effective means of gradually rebuilding their sexual relationship and of tackling their specific sexual problems. The second is to clarify the nature and causes of the couple's sexual problems. Most couples encounter difficulties at some stage of therapy, and a cardinal rule is to regard such difficulties as a source of specific clues about the causes of the couple's problems. The therapist's task at such times is to help the couple understand that this provides a chance for valuable learning, and then to help them explore the reasons for the difficulty in order that they can make further progress. This is the most skilful part of therapy. Because of its importance, the second part of this chapter is devoted to detailed discussion of the strategies that therapists may use in order to facilitate the progress of couples in therapy and to help couples understand the reasons for any difficulties they encounter.

When general relationship issues become apparent, other approaches, which are discussed in Chapter 11, may be necessary.

THE NATURE OF THE THERAPEUTIC RELATIONSHIP IN SEX THERAPY

When couples first seek help for sexual problems they usually feel very vulnerable because they are exposing to a stranger some of the most private aspects of their relationship, and they are having to admit to failure. The trust and respect that should develop between a couple and their therapist early in therapy is an important influence on how a couple engage in the treatment programme.

Some couples are very dependent on the therapist at the beginning of treatment. This is not necessarily harmful to the therapeutic process. The therapist should encourage the couple to gradually accept responsibility for their problems and should emphasize that the eventual outcome will largely depend on their own efforts. As treatment proceeds, the solution to problems should increasingly become the responsibility of the couple. During successful treatment, couples become less and less dependent on the therapist until the time arrives when they feel happy to leave the treatment programme. However, some couples offer profound resistance to this shift, and continually try to provoke an authoritarian response from the therapist, thus emphasizing their dependency and helplessness. Unless this situation is confronted it can prove a major obstacle to successful treatment.

When a therapist becomes aware that the relationship with a couple has developed in this way, several strategies are available, including the following. First, the couple can be firmly reminded of the need for them to take responsibility for themselves and to be prepared to seek their own explanation for, and solutions to, their failures. Secondly, they may need to be reminded of the time-limited nature of the therapeutic contact (p. 192) as a means of emphasizing this point. Thirdly, for a couple who are sufficiently sophisticated to be able to examine the nature of the therapeutic relationship, the therapist could explain to them what appears to be happening. The best approach, however, is for the therapist to avoid being drawn into this situation in the first place, by reflecting back questions and requiring the couple to make decisions for themselves.

Nevertheless, it is important to recognize that there may be times when it seems appropriate to allow a couple to be relatively dependent. This may happen, for example, when a couple have had a very distressing experience and require maximum support and encouragement from the therapist.

Some couples form a very different relationship with the therapist, and offer considerable resistance to the therapist's suggestions. It is often one rather than both partners who behaves in this way. This kind of interaction may develop because of excessive anxiety about receiving help. Another common reason is that one partner feels extremely insecure about his or her sexuality. Refusal to engage constructively in the therapy programme is a means of preventing this insecurity being confronted and explored. The therapist should explain to the couple what appears to be happening, before this pattern has become established.

There are several other important general characteristics of the therapeutic relationship in sex therapy which may contribute to the success or failure of treatment. These all apply to some extent to any therapy based on psychological principles. We shall briefly consider some ways in which a therapist can enhance the quality of the therapeutic relationship with regard to each of these factors.

Empathic understanding

The therapist should not only try to understand a couple's problems in terms of, for example, causal factors, but should also communicate to the couple recognition of the distress they are experiencing through comments such as : 'I can see how distressing the problem is for you both'; 'It must have taken a lot of courage to come and seek help'. Such simple statements provide considerable relief for many couples and may make it easier for them to engage in therapy.

Warmth and caring

The therapeutic relationship should not be distant and cold. The warmth of the relationship can be enhanced if the therapist adopts a generally friendly manner, and comments on events in the life of a couple other than solely those in their sexual relationship. The therapist might enquire, for example, how a special outing went, or how a child is getting on preparing for an examination.

However, protracted discussion of matters which are not directly relevant to treatment should be avoided. The couple should also be aware that the therapist cares what happens to them, both when progress is being made and when difficulties have been encountered. However, when the couple report poor progress it is important that, after demonstrating concern, the therapist then adopts a positive stance and emphasizes how such experiences should be used to learn more about the problem and ways of overcoming it. The therapist might, for example, say: 'I am sorry to hear that things did not go well this week—that must have been disappointing for you. Let us look more closely at precisely what happened so that we can try to find the reasons for it. This may help clarify what you now need to do in order to prevent the same thing happening next week'.

Trust

Clearly it is vital that couples who are receiving help for sexual problems should trust their therapists. In particular they must feel confident that what they say is absolutely confidential at all times. This should be explained at the outset. Some couples may be concerned about the treatment notes that therapists keep, and what might happen to such notes. It should be explained that it is necessary to keep notes in order to provide a record of what has happened at various stages in treatment, and to remind both the therapist and the couple what homework assignments had been planned each week (medical and other health service practitioners must also keep for medico-legal purposes). Therapists should reassure couples that the notes will be kept under the strictest security.

Couples also need to develop such trust in their therapist that eventually they will feel able, if necessary, to reveal their weaknesses, fears, and special concerns, such as those concerning sexual fantasies they regard as taboo, or anxieties about the usefulness of the treatment approach. This type of trust often only develops after several treatment sessions.

Respect

Therapists should ensure that they show respect for couples by emphasizing that they recognize that their problem is special for them, and by dealing with them as responsible adults with valid ideas about their own problem. Furthermore, treatment programmes should be designed in keeping with each couple's sexual value system. Special care is particularly necessary when organizing treatment for older couples and those from other cultures, for whom some forms of sexual behaviour will be totally unacceptable.

Encouragement and support

There are many ways in which therapists can be encouraging and supportive during sex therapy. For example, they can express pleasure and offer appropriate praise when couples report progress. When a couple encounter problems it should be made clear that these are to be expected and that therapy is about helping couples surmount such difficulties. When a couple express the fear that they are not getting anywhere with solving their problems they should be reminded of the gains they have made so far, however small these might be.

Instillation of hope

Throughout treatment, therapists should do all they can to maintain a hopeful attitude concerning the ability of couples to surmount their difficulties. The right atmosphere can be established when presenting the formulation of a couple's problem (Chapter 7) by pointing out the strengths of each partner, such as their motivation; by emphasizing the positive aspects of both their sexual relationship and their general relationship (e.g. affection, mutual interests, communication); and by indicating the early benefits which therapy is likely to bring. During treatment the therapist can express confidence in the likely outcome. However, a therapist should only express appropriate confidence. Apart from being misleading, an over-confident approach can make a couple uneasy, and, if the eventual outcome is poor, can make termination of treatment extremely difficult.

HOW TO HELP COUPLES WHEN THEY
ENCOUNTER DIFFICULTIES

Occasionally, there is a successful outcome from sex therapy with an entirely behavioural and educational approach. The majority of couples, however, encounter difficulties at one or more stages during therapy. This section concerns how such difficulties manifest themselves, and what therapists can do to help couples overcome them.

Difficulties may occur at any stage of treatment. The timing of these is not arbitrary, but can usually be explained by the nature of the presenting problem and its causes.

Difficulties early in treatment

Early difficulties may present in several ways, including the following:

1. *Failure to have homework sessions.* A couple may return to the therapist after the first week in which they intended to begin sensate focus, or after each of several initial weeks, saying they have not managed to have any homework sessions. The couple may provide excuses such as being too busy, too tired, having invited relatives to stay, or simply having forgotten. It is also surprising how often couples develop minor illness during the first week or two of therapy.

2. *Negative experiences.* Some couples will have had sessions of sensate focus, but report only negative experiences. These include, for example, getting tense, being ticklish, thinking about other things, feeling embarrassed, or even feeling nothing at all.

3. *Neutral experiences.* Some couples will say that they have learnt nothing new, or that they have done it all before.

4. *Obstructive behaviour.* A couple may report what appears to have been obstructive behaviour on the part of one or both of them, e.g. repeatedly causing arguments and therefore creating the wrong atmosphere for the homework sessions, one partner jeering at the other partner's attempts to begin caressing, or repeatedly falling asleep.

5. *Breaking the ban on sexual intercourse.* This is very common.

6. *Only one partner arriving for a treatment session.* This can occur at any stage during treatment, but is especially likely early on. Although there may be a perfectly acceptable explanation for this, it often indicates a serious difficulty.

Early difficulties may be encountered in the treatment of any type of sexual dysfunction, but seem to occur more often when the problem is secondary impairment of sexual interest or erectile dysfunction. Sometimes a couple fail to get started on the programme because of chronic ill-feeling resulting from years of experiencing a poor sexual relationship. For example, a woman who had endured years of frustration because her partner did not bother with foreplay before sexual intercourse needed to air her resentment before she could begin the homework sessions. Early difficulties are particularly likely when a couple have problems in their general relationship. When early difficulties occur, the therapist should always reconsider the initial assessment of the couple's general relationship in case something has been missed.

Difficulties in the middle of treatment

Many couples make good initial progress but then encounter difficulties in the middle of therapy. The following are examples of how difficulties at this stage may present:

1. *A couple cease having homework sessions.* This often occurs when a couple move from non-genital to genital sensate focus.

2. *The sessions cease being pleasurable.* This often indicates that one partner has started to get tense during, or at the prospect of, the homework sessions.

3. *Breaking the ban on sexual intercourse.* Again, this is common.

Difficulties in mid-therapy may occur in the treatment of any type of sexual dysfunction, but are particularly likely when the dysfunction results from fear of intimacy (p. 71); generalized sexual anxiety or inhibition; one partner's specific aversion to the genitals of the other; one partner's feelings of inadequacy or distaste concerning his or her own genitals; and fear of arousal (including not trusting the partner to keep to the agreed limits of sexual activity). Some couples have difficulty because of fear on the part of one, or even both of them, concerning the next stage of the programme. A woman who has vaginismus, for example, may find genital sensate focus difficult because she knows that some form of vaginal penetration will be suggested next. Breaking the ban on sexual intercourse sometimes occurs when one partner finds the intimacy of genital sensate focus difficult. Sexual intercourse both helps avoid the problem and effectively terminates sexual activity.

Difficulties late in treatment

Difficulties towards the end of treatment, such as at the stage of vaginal containment, often result either from fear of failure (e.g. men with erectile dysfunction), or from fear of success. The latter may occur because a couple recognize that successful completion of the final stages will herald the end of treatment, and they fear that without the therapist's support they might not be able to sustain the progress they have made. Gradual termination of treatment and discussion of the fear are usually sufficient to resolve this type of problem (p. 193).

What to do when difficulties occur

1. *Check that the couple have understood the instructions.* Before assuming that a couple have actually encountered difficulty the therapist should check that the instructions were clearly understood. Misunderstandings in sex therapy are quite common, but can mostly be avoided by establishing beforehand that a couple fully understand their homework assignments, and, if necessary, writing the instructions down.

2. *Find out what happened.* The therapist should obtain a detailed account of any sessions the couple have had, or any attempts by either partner to initiate sessions. If the latter has not occurred the therapist should discuss what each partner has thought and felt about this.

3. *Assess how serious the problem is.* If the difficulty has not been the result of misunderstanding, the therapist should consider how serious it appears to be. Many difficulties are relatively *minor*; for example, finding the initial sensate focus sessions awkward or artificial, feeling embarrassed at being naked, or the partners not inviting each other for sessions in the way that had been suggested. Such problems are more common during the early part of the programme. Quite often, however, it will become obvious that a couple have encountered a *major* difficulty, possibly one associated with the main cause of their presenting problem. The management of these two types of difficulties will be considered separately.

The management of minor difficulties. This is often straightforward. The following are strategies the therapist can use (Table 9.1):

1. *Acknowledge difficulty and offer encouragement.* It is often sufficient for the therapist to say to a couple that he or she recognizes that they have encountered some difficulty, and then to explain that many couples experience similar difficulties at this stage but that these soon disappear with more practice. This would be the approach to use, for example, when a couple report that their initial sensate focus sessions lacked spontaneity, or were a little embarrassing. The therapist might also emphasize how important it is for a couple to work at solving their sexual problem and how this necessitates careful planning (which may reduce spontaneity) and a less inhibited approach to sexuality (which might initially cause embarrassment).

2. *Suggest easier or alternative homework assignments.* It will sometimes be apparent that a couple's current homework assignment is too difficult and poses too great a demand on them. The assignment might then be broken down into smaller steps. For example, if one partner strongly dislikes being naked the therapist might agree that some clothing (e.g. a nightdress) could initially be worn. If a phobic problem has become apparent, as in the case of a woman who becomes tense if her breasts are caressed, the therapist might suggest a graded approach, as described in the

TABLE 9.1

Strategies which may facilitate progress in sex therapy

Strategies for minor difficulties

1. Acknowledge difficulty and offer encouragement
2. Suggest easier or alternative homework assignments

Strategies for major difficulties

1. Identify negative thoughts and attitudes
2. Interpretation
3. Explore a series of explanations

Other useful strategies

1. Identify the positive benefits of homework assignments
2. Attribute positive intentions to actions
3. Positive relabelling
4. Reassurance about 'normality' of experiences
5. Giving permission
6. Paradoxical intention
7. Seeing the partners individually
8. Confrontation

previous chapter (p. 146). Sometimes the therapist will need to suggest an alternative approach. For example, in treating a man with premature ejaculation it might be found that when the man is being caressed by his partner he cannot identify when his level of sexual arousal has reached the point beyond which ejaculation is inevitable. The therapist might suggest that for a limited period the man should concentrate on stimulating himself to ejaculation, either in the presence of his partner or alone (p. 221).

The management of more serious difficulties. When a couple get into difficulties, both they and their therapist may be unclear why this has happened. In some cases the therapist may understand why the difficulty has occurred, perhaps even having predicted it on the basis of the assessment. In either case, the therapist should try to help the partners understand the difficulty, because they may then be able to approach their homework assignments with a new resolve. Alternatively, once the difficulty has been understood, it may become apparent that a different approach is needed. Sometimes, of course, it will become obvious that the couple's problems are not amenable to sex therapy.

Three strategies that can be used when couples encounter major difficulties during sex therapy are discussed below.

1. *Identify negative thoughts and attitudes.* It was noted above that when a couple report having been unable to carry out their homework assignments, or having had a very negative experience, the therapist's first task is to obtain from both partners a clear and detailed description of what actually happened. In their accounts they should be asked to describe any thoughts or feelings evoked by the assignment (including actually trying it or just contemplating it). Each partner should then be asked for any explanation that he or she has for the difficulty. If either the partners or therapist (or all three) are unclear why the difficulty has occurred, the following approach is often helpful. It is derived from the congnitive therapy approach to depression proposed by Beck and his colleagues (Beck *et al.* 1979).

A negative response to a homework assignment can be understood in terms of a model (shown diagramatically in Fig. 9.1) which includes the following three factors:

    (i) immediate *negative thoughts* or *images* that are evoked by the homework assignment;

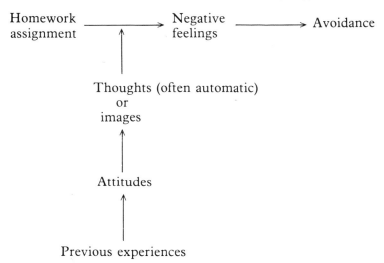

Fig. 9.1 A cognitive model useful in explaining negative responses to homework assignments

(ii) *attitudes* that conflict with the homework assignment (and which generate the negative thoughts or images);

(iii) *previous experiences* which have shaped a person's attitudes towards sexuality.

This model is illustrated by the following two examples of women who had difficulty when instructed to begin genital sensate focus.

A woman who had primary impairment of sexual interest became very tense at this stage. The immediate thought she experienced when her husband began genital caressing was 'this is revolting'. The attitude which explained this thought was that she believed that her genitals were an unpleasant part of her body. The previous experience related to this attitude was that from the age of nine until she was 14 her father had repeatedly fondled her genitals. At first she had enjoyed this, but later, when she realized it was wrong, she had felt disgusted.

Another woman stopped the homework sessions when her husband tried to caress her genitals because she had an image of herself looking stupid and repulsive if she abandoned herself to sexual arousal, and thought her partner would regard her in the same way. This image arose out of her very negative general attitudes towards her sexuality, especially her genital anatomy. This attitude had developed when at the age of 19 it had been discovered that she had a serious abnormality of her vagina which necessitated reconstructive surgery.

Unfortunately, the explanations for major difficulties are often not as immediately clear as they were in these couples. One reason is that the negative thoughts which are evoked by a homework assignment are often 'automatic' (Fig. 9.1). In other words, they are overlearned habits of thinking of which the person may not be clearly aware because they are very fleeting, rather than being carefully considered ideas. Similarly, a person's attitudes towards sexuality may not be fully apparent either to that person or to others. The experiences upon which attitudes are based, especially those that have occurred early in a person's life, are often obscure.

The therapist should first explain that negative reactions to a homework assignment are usually based on thoughts or images evoked by what has been suggested, and that identification of these can often help uncover important attitudes towards sexuality (i.e. this can be explained on the basis of Fig. 9.1). The first step is to identify the thoughts and images. One approach is to suggest that the person who is responding negatively to an assignment notes down after a session (or after avoiding one) any thoughts or images that have occurred.

Couples very often find it difficult to identify automatic thoughts or images without assistance. The therapist can help by encouraging them to explore a series of possible thoughts of images as described below (p. 165). In order to increase the couple's understanding the therapist might also attempt to relate the thoughts or images and attitudes to earlier experiences. Fortunately, successful therapy is usually possible even when the original cause of a negative attitude remains obscure. Nevertheless, new information about early experiences is sometimes recalled during such exploration, or, if having been knowingly withheld by one of the partners, is eventually revealed (e.g. anxieties about homosexual experiences).

Sex therapy sometimes highlights a deeply ingrained attitude or other psychological problem in one partner which seems resistant to any form of brief intervention. This may occur with problems of intimacy, or those involving low self-esteem. Under such circumstances the therapist should consider whether referral for some other type of help, such as individual psychotherapy, is indicated.

It is totally inappropriate for a person to be in both psychotherapy and sex therapy at the same time. However, if psychotherapy is successful, further sex therapy may help a couple to benefit more from the gains made through individual psychotherapy.

2. *Interpretation.* When a therapist thinks he or she has a reasonable understanding of why a couple have encountered difficulties, this explanation might be discussed with the couple. Interpretations include explanations at various levels, as indicated in Fig. 9.1. For example, they may be explanations concerning current thoughts or attitudes, or concerning experiences which have occurred much earlier in a person's life.

An example of the former was an interpretation provided for a man who was withholding from pleasuring his partner. The therapist said: 'I think that maybe the reason why you won't caress your partner in the way she wants you to is because you know this would be likely to arouse her and you are worried that if she starts to get a lot of pleasure from sex she might seek out another partner'.

An example of an interpretation linking an early experience with current behaviour for a similar case was as follows: 'I think the reason you find it difficult to caress your wife and help her to become aroused is that, because of the close relationship with your mother, you have always tended unconsciously to divide women into those who are sexually active and responsive, and therefore 'immoral' and those who are modest about sexuality, but who fit more into your concept of an appropriate wife and mother. In other words, you find it difficult to accept that your partner can be both your wife, and also be a highly sexually responsive woman.'

In sex therapy it is usually preferable to avoid interpretations of this kind, partly because an interpretation unacceptable to the couple can undermine their confidence in the therapist. Interpretations should be offered as tentative hypotheses to be evaluated by the couple, in line with the general sex therapy approach. Inexperienced therapists are sometimes too ready to offer interpretations, and also tend to do so too early in therapy, in which case rejection of an interpretation by a couple is more likely.

3. *Explore a series of explanations.* This is recommended as a better strategy, especially for the relatively inexperienced therapist. It has an important advantage over the interpretative approach in that it encourages couples themselves to be more active in seeking explanations for their difficulties. It can be used to help

a couple identify negative thoughts and attitudes which are causing the difficulties.

First, the therapist thinks of a range of possible explanations for the couple's current problem. These are then presented to the couple, the therapist making it clear to them that these are only possibilities, not facts. The therapist then helps the partners to consider each explanation in turn in order to determine which is the most likely. It is preferable if at least one of the proferred explanations is a highly improbable one, easily rejected by the couple. This may enhance the couple's involvement in exploring other more likely possibilities. Once a likely explanation is found this in itself may allow a couple to resume their progress, or it may clearly indicate what therapeutic strategies are now appropriate. The following two examples illustrate this procedure:

A couple were in sex therapy because of the man's erectile difficulties. When the couple moved on to the stage of genital sensate focus the man's wife failed to touch her partner's penis in spite of agreeing that she would do this. It was unclear to both the couple and the therapist why she had this difficulty. The therapist therefore offered the couple a series of possible explanations, as follows, for the couple to consider:
(i) the wife had not stroked her partner's penis because she did not know how to do it;
(ii) she thought she might hurt him;
(iii) she thought she would find it unpleasant;
(iv) she thought it was a 'dirty' thing to do;
(v) she was worried that if her husband got an erection he would want to have sexual intercourse;
(vi) she did not want to help him;
(vii) she did not want to give him pleasure.
The wife immediately rejected the sixth possibility, insisting she was very keen that they should overcome their problem. The therapist then helped the couple to consider each of the other possibilities in turn. Eventually it became clear that the wife's main concerns were she did not know how best to stimulate her husband and also that she feared she might hurt him. This led to a discussion of how her husband could show her how he liked being caressed.

A couple had entered sex therapy because the wife had lacked interest in sex for the previous four years. During each of the first three weeks of treatment her husband had failed to invite her to have any sessions of non-genital sensate focus. The couple were unable to explain this, so the therapist suggested the following possible explanations:

(i) the husband might still be angry and resentful about his wife having been unresponsive for so long;
(ii) he feared close sexual involvement;
(iii) he did not want his wife to overcome the problem in case she became sexually too demanding;
(iv) he would not be able to caress her in a way that would give her pleasure;
(v) he would not be able to control himself and would force her to have sexual intercourse;
(vi) he feared she might get sexually aroused and be unable to control herself.

Both partners denied the fourth possibility because the husband had been able to give his wife a great deal of pleasure before the problem began. After consideration of all the other possibilities the husband thought that his long-standing resentment was the most likely explanation. He was then helped to air this resentment.

Thoughts and attitudes which are likely to cause difficulties and prevent progress can be grouped into those concerning (a) the nature of an assignment; (b) the possible consequences of carrying out the assignment; and, (c) others, which cannot be easily classified. Examples of thoughts and attitudes in each of these categories include the following:

(a) *Concerning the nature of a homework assignment*: that it is 'wrong', unpleasant, unhelpful, or too difficult.

(b) *Concerning the consequences*: fear of failure, of being hurt, of being exposed as inadequate, of being taken advantage of, of becoming emotionally close, of being abandoned when aroused, of evoking the partner's disapproval, of being ridiculed, of becoming pregnant, and of losing control.

(c) *Others*: wishing to avoid possible failure, needing to maintain power over a dysfunctional partner, or to get back at the partner, and feeling angry or resentful because of other problems in the relationship.

As noted above, helping a couple to understand why they have encountered difficulties is quite often sufficient to enable them to approach their homework assignments afresh and with greater chance of success. However, as discussed below, there are several other strategies which can be used to initiate progress.

Other useful strategies. In this section, several other strategies which can be used to mobilize a couple's enthusiasm to overcome their difficulties and to progress in therapy are considered (Table 9.1). Most of these strategies are intended to help couples to focus on the positive aspects of their relationship and on their efforts and their experiences during therapy. A good general principle for therapists is to *be positive and to avoid being drawn into repeated discussions of failure, and, even when failures keep occurring, to focus on the positive aspects of these experiences.*

1. *Identify the positive benefits of homework assignments.* When a couple are apprehensive about a homework assignment, the therapist should ask them to consider how they might benefit if they were to try what has been suggested. For example, partners who think they will find it difficult to let each other know how they are feeling during their pleasuring sessions should be asked to consider what each would gain from being able to let the other know what he or she likes and dislikes.

2. *Attribute positive intentions to actions.* When a couple have not kept precisely to the therapist's instructions, it is sometimes appropriate and helpful to interpret this in a positive fashion. For example, if one person has been over-demanding, such as by asking for homework sessions out of turn, the therapist might interpret this as being the result of enthusiasm and attraction to the partner. However, the therapist should also remind the couple of the reasons for the original instructions.

3. *Positive relabelling.* This consists of trying, whenever possible, to reframe in a positive light events which a couple view negatively or as a failure. The following two examples should make this clear.

A couple repeatedly announced at the beginning of their treatment sessions that they had had a 'poor week'. The therapist's response was, 'I'm sorry to hear that, but what were the best things that happened?' On another occasion, when one partner reported that a specific assignment did not go well, the therapist asked: 'what were the things that you *liked* about it?'.

A man receiving treatment for erectile dysfunction thought that his loss of erection during genital sensate focus was a disaster. The therapist first responded by encouraging him to acknowledge the progress he had made in therapy so far, in that at least he was now able to get an erection, and then asked him what was so catastrophic about his losing his erection since he and his partner were still able to provide each other with pleasure irrespective of whether or not he had one.

When a couple report that things have not gone well, or that they have encountered a specific problem, the therapist should emphasize that sex therapy is a learning process, and that often the best way to learn is through mistakes or difficulties. This is especially important early in treatment when a couple may have unrealistic expectations of early success and hence be unreasonably disappointed if things do not go well.

4. *Reassurance about 'normality' of experiences.* It is often appropriate for the therapist to reassure a couple (or one partner) that some aspect of their sexual experience or behaviour is perfectly normal in the sense that it is in keeping with the experience or behaviour of many other people. This may be particularly helpful when discussing topics such as sexual fantasies, oral sex, or the frequency of sexual activity. Some couples think that their behaviour or experience is in some way perverse, or at least very different from that of most of the rest of the general population; the therapist's reassurance that this is not so may help them to enjoy their sexual relationship more freely.

5. *Giving permission.* In suggesting homework assignments necessary to help couples resolve their sexual difficulties, therapists are often effectively giving people permission to engage in sexual behaviour that they might previously never have considered, or never liked to suggest to their partners. Sometimes, the therapist's suggestions are in sharp contrast to the attitudes towards sexuality which were encouraged in either or both partners during their upbringing.

For example, a couple were in therapy because the woman had primary impaired sexual interest resulting from clear messages from her mother that sexual activity was something to be endured under sufferance in order to gain other benefits from a relationship. After discussing the woman's right to enjoy sexual arousal, the therapist encouraged her to begin to focus on any pleasant sensations she could get from being caressed.

The permission-giving role of the therapist, which is often a powerful one, brings with it a most important need for caution. Therapists must always guard against imposing values on couples by encouraging sexual behaviour which they will not only find unacceptable, but which is not essential in terms of the problems with which they presented. After describing a new homework assignment the therapist should therefore inquire whether the couple are happy to try it. If they are not, the reasons for this should be explored. If the couple still do not find the suggestion acceptable the therapist must consider whether there are any other means of helping them to achieve their chosen goals. If there do not appear to be any, this should be explained to the couple.

6. *Paradoxical intention.* Sometimes a therapist will make a suggestion to a couple which at first appears contrary to the goal of therapy, but which the therapist suspects might actually facilitate progress. For example, when a couple have been striving unsuccessfully to arouse each other it is often very helpful to suggest that instead they should try deliberately to avoid arousal. The aim here would be to remove the couple's self-induced pressure because this might enable them to enjoy their caressing in a more relaxed fashion and therefore eventually become aroused. Similarly, in the treatment of a man with erectile dysfunction who has considerable performance anxieties the therapist might suggest that the man tries to avoid getting an erection, and instead concentrates solely on pleasurable sensations given and received during sensate focus.

7. *Seeing the partners individually.* Although in sex therapy one tries as far as possible to conduct all treatment sessions with both partners together, it sometimes becomes important to see the partners separately for at least one session. The usual reason is that unexplained difficulties have arisen, and the therapist believes that one of the partners may have the answer but is unwilling to disclose it in front of the other partner. For example, in an individual session, a woman might reveal that she has always faked orgasm but did not know how to let her partner know this.

Sometimes this strategy will uncover an affair by one partner, in which case the therapist must explain that sex therapy cannot be continued while the affair lasts. This raises a difficult issue concerning confidentiality. The therapist must make it clear that the affair will not be revealed to the other partner; in the subsequent conjoint session the therapist will have to use some nonspecific excuse for ending therapy.

8. *Confrontation.* When a therapist has failed to help a couple using the approaches which seemed most likely to help them, and there is no obvious reason for this (such as a poor general

relationship), confronting them with the discrepancy between their stated goals and their actual behaviour can sometimes mobilize greater motivation. This might be the case, for example, with a couple who attend treatment sessions for several weeks but never find time for homework sessions. Once a couple have been confronted in this way it is often wise to agree a set number of further sessions, usually between two and four, following which treatment will be terminated if there has been no further progress. It is usually better to terminate treatment relatively soon after it becomes clear that the outcome is likely to be poor, rather than encourage a couple to continue for many more sessions in the vain hope of success. Prolonged treatment may only result in demoralization for both the couple and the therapist.

CONCLUSIONS

The general nature of the therapeutic relationship between the therapist and a couple is often important in determining outcome. Attention to specific features of this relationship can enhance the therapeutic process. The balance of the relationship usually changes as treatment proceeds, with most couples gradually moving away from relative dependency on the therapist to greater autonomy, until eventually they feel able to leave the treatment programme. If it becomes apparent that this shift in the nature of the relationship is not happening when it perhaps should, the therapist may have to explore why this is so. Some couples pose the opposite problem, offering profound resistance to the therapist's suggestions. Once recognized, this problem should also be explored as soon as possible.

Difficulties during treatment are to be expected, and usually offer the best opportunities to clarify the reasons for a couple's sexual problems. Difficulties may occur at various stages in the programme and their timing often reflects the nature of the sexual problem. Minor difficulties are usually easily overcome. Major difficulties require careful exploration. Various ways of doing this, including a cognitive approach, have been discussed. In addition, there are various other strategies which can enhance the therapeutic process and these have been considered together with examples of their application.

10

Educational aspects

In Chapter 5 it was emphasized that inadequate or inaccurate information about sexuality may contribute to the development and maintenance of sexual dysfunction. Provision of accurate, sensible information is therefore an important component of treatment. In order to be able to do this the therapist must have a reasonable knowledge of sexual anatomy and sexual response. Although Chapter 2 of this book contains some of the more important facts relevant to sex therapy, trainee therapists are also recommended to read one of the more detailed texts (e.g Masters and Johnson 1966; Bancroft 1983).

The educational process often begins during the initial assessment and formulation, and continues throughout therapy as a couple raise questions about aspects of sexuality which are a source of concern. However, this component of the therapeutic programme should not rely solely on the couple asking questions; special attention to facts about sexuality should be built into the programme. There are two means of doing this, both of which are recommended in the treatment of *all* couples.

The first is to ask the couple to read a suitable book about sexuality. For several years we have recommended Delvin's (1974) *Book of love* and found this acceptable and of help to most couples. Several alternatives are available. The therapist must have read any such book beforehand. The point at which one suggests such reading depends on the nature of a couple's problems and also their progress. Generally we recommend it just before, or at the same time as, the 'educational session' (see below). Some therapists may feel they ought to lend couples reading material, but probably it is better to ask them to buy it themselves, provided they can afford it. How they go about this task can itself provide useful information. The couple will also be able to refer to it at other times. It is worthwhile checking which local bookshops have it available, or how it can be obtained by post. The couple should be shown a copy of the book before being asked to buy it.

The second, and complementary way of ensuring that a couple have a satisfactory understanding of sexual anatomy and sexual response is by devoting part or all of one treatment session to this purpose. This can be done in a relatively didactic fashion, while allowing plenty of opportunity for the partners to ask questions. We call this part of the programme the *educational session*.

THE EDUCATIONAL SESSION

With some couples, special attention must be paid to improving their knowledge about sexuality at the beginning of therapy. These include couples whose sexual information is so poor that they lack the confidence to approach each other sexually. However, in most cases the educational session should occur later in treatment, especially as there is so much else the therapist needs to cover at the beginning. Clinical experience suggests that the most appropriate time is somewhere between the third and the sixth session of treatment, usually just before, or just after, the couple begin the genital sensate focus part of the programme.

The aims of the education session are essentially threefold:
(1) to provide information and dispel sexual myths in a way that will help a couple improve their sexual technique;
(2) to alleviate anxieties and enhance confidence;
(3) to identify any important blindspots or fallacies that may be contributing to a couple's difficulties.

The educational session need not take long; 20-30 minutes is usually enough. As has been emphasized elsewhere in this book with regard to providing information, it is essential that the therapist keeps things as simple as possible and does not overload the couple with facts. If necessary, this educational input can be spread across two treatment sessions.

For the sake of clarity, pictures should be used in the education session. A couple's reactions to them can sometimes be informative. Occasionally, pictures can also be a useful means of desensitization. The therapist should find a book which contains appropriate pictures, or else obtain photographs and drawings which can be kept in a folio and used for this purpose. Some therapists use slides which they project in their office. Although diagrams can help in clarifying the nature of sexual anatomy, it is also recommended that photographs of actual people and sexual anatomy are used.

A collection of pictures which will usually be sufficient for the educational session includes the following:

(1) a full (head to feet) view of a naked man and woman;
(2) female external genitals in which the vaginal entrance, labia, and clitoris are shown;
(3) internal anatomy of the female genitals (simple diagram);
(4) male external genitals showing the penis, glans, scrotum, and testis;
(5) internal anatomy of the male genitals (simple diagram).

In addition, diagrams in the form of graphs showing the stages of sexual response (Figs 2.3 and 2.7) may be useful, although many therapists prefer to draw these themselves during the session. Other pictures or diagrams which can be used with some couples are the following: female breast, changes in female internal genitals during the stages of sexual response, and male genitals with the penis erect.

Throughout the educational session the therapist should emphasize the similarities as well as the differences between the sexual anatomy and responses of a man and a woman. Discovery of the similarities between the sexes, particularly in terms of sexual response, is a helpful revelation for some couples. The variability in response that the same individual is likely to experience at different times should also be stressed. The therapist should ensure that the session is as relevant as possible to each couple, providing information that is likely to be helpful with regard to their particular problems and needs. Special care should be paid to terminology. Technical jargon should be avoided whenever possible, and, when this is difficult, the therapist must explain how a technical term (e.g. 'ejaculation' or 'orgasm') is equivalent to a term in more common general use (e.g. 'coming'). The couple should be encouraged to ask questions.

In the educational session, first one sex and then the other should be considered; usually it is arbitrary which is considered first. For both sexes, the therapist should begin by describing sexual anatomy and then sexual response. Here, female sexual anatomy and response will be considered first. The range of topics covered in the rest of this chapter is far more extensive than would be included in the educational session with any one couple. The therapist should choose the topics relevant to each couple.

THE WOMAN

Sexual anatomy

The therapist might begin by showing the couple a picture of a woman's general anatomy, emphasizing that a certain amount of asymmetry (e.g. of the breasts, shoulder height) is normal. At this point a picture of a man's general anatomy can be shown, or, even better, a picture showing a man and woman side by side, in order that the woman's form can be compared with that of the man. The therapist should emphasize the wide variation in body build and shape of both women and men, and how confidence about one's body can be an important factor in enjoying sex with a partner.

A picture of a woman's external genitals should then be shown, and the following pointed out: the vaginal entrance, labia minora and majora, clitoris (with explanation that in terms of anatomy and sensitivity it is equivalent to the glans penis), clitoral hood, urethral opening, mons pubis, and pubic hair. The wide variation in the appearance of the female genitals among different women should be explained, because some women are concerned that their genitals appear different from those in books.

The couple might also be shown a simple diagram of a woman's internal genital anatomy, and the therapist can indicate: the nature of the inside of the vagina (explaining that when empty and the woman unaroused the sides are touching each other, but that it has considerable potential to expand and also, in its outer third, to 'grasp' the penis); the uterus, and cervix (feels like the tip of the nose if touched with finger). It is important to stress that the most sensitive parts of the woman's genitals are the clitoris and entrance to the vagina, and that inside the vagina there is little sensation except to pressure. This surprises many men who have assumed that what a woman most enjoys in fore-play is deep vaginal stimulation. However, in view of recent work suggesting that part of the anterior wall of the vagina may be highly sensitive, one should mention the possibility that the woman may enjoy gentle stimulation to this region.

Sexual response

In describing sexual arousal it is helpful to use the graphs of the stages of sexual response (Fig. 2.3), either showing the couple the complete graphs or, preferably, drawing them (having established that the couple understand how a simple graph is constructed).

While reading the next section, and when deciding what to include in this part of the educational session with a couple, the therapist may find it helpful to refer to Table 2.1.

Excitement.   First, the therapist should explain that the process of sexual arousal is exactly the same, irrespective of the means of stimulation. Thus the same responses may occur when a woman is being caressed by a partner, reading an erotic book, having a sexual fantasy, or watching an erotic film. Many of the changes during sexual arousal are the result of increased blood flow to the genitals and breasts.

The specific anatomical changes which occur during sexual arousal might be described as follows. *Vaginal lubrication*, which occurs very soon after the start of sexual stimulation, is rather like 'sweating' of the vaginal wall, and occurs inside the vagina. Some men look for wetness at the entrance to the vagina as a sign of arousal. If this is not apparent they may incorrectly assume that their partner is not aroused. The moisture may not reach the entrance to the vagina until the woman has been aroused for some time, unless a finger is inserted into the vagina. The *clitoris* enlarges early in sexual arousal. It may be so sensitive that for a while a woman finds direct contact with the clitoral head painful, preferring indirect clitoral stimulation, or stimulation confined to the clitoral shaft. Massage of the clitoral head may be appreciated more when arousal has increased. A *skin flush* may appear across the upper part of the body as arousal increases, but not in all women and not on every occasion. Similarly, *nipple erection* and *breast enlargement* do not occur in all women.

It can be very helpful, especially for a woman who has difficulty in becoming aroused, to explain how the subjective experience of sexual excitement consists of waves of arousal, and that when a woman feels such a wave fading away it does not mean that her arousal is diminishing. Provided she does not become anxious, with continuing foreplay she should experience further similar waves of arousal which will gradually increase in intensity. This contrasts with a man who, although having similar subjective experiences of arousal, can rely on erection as an obvious sign of continuing sexual arousal.

Plateau. The therapist should emphasize that this is not a direct stage of sexual arousal, but that there are some particular features which accompany very high arousal. First, there is often a considerable increase in muscle tension which may be obvious in movements of the body and facial grimacing. This tension heralds orgasm in many women. Secondly, ballooning of the inner two-thirds of the vagina is sometimes apparent to the woman's partner. Swelling of the outer third of the vagina (the 'orgasmic platform') ensures continuing stimulation of the penis. Thirdly, retraction of the clitoris under the clitoral hood can sometimes mislead a man into thinking his partner is no longer aroused.

Orgasm. The therapist should explain that orgasm consists of both subjective sensations and contractions of the muscles of the pelvis. The intensity of orgasm will vary greatly from one occasion to another and some women are not aware of muscle contractions. It should be emphasized that the nature of an orgasm is essentially the same, irrespective of whether it occurs through direct clitoral stimulation, or through the indirect stimulation which occurs with sexual intercourse in most positions, unless the woman is receiving additional manual stimulation. Thus the myth that there are different types of orgasms, clitoral and vaginal, should be firmly quashed. The therapist might explain how the clitoris can be indirectly stimulated during sexual intercourse, by the stretching of bands of tissue extending from the vaginal entrance to the clitoris via the labia minora, and how in certain positions, direct stimulation from the man's penis is possible. For the woman who has difficulty in experiencing orgasm during sexual intercourse, with or without stimulation of the clitoris, it is most important that the therapist explains the wide range of orgasmic responsivity among normal women (p. 14).

Resolution. The therapist can now describe how all the changes that occurred during sexual arousal gradually revert to normal following orgasm (or after cessation of stimulation when orgasm has now occurred). The importance of this phase, when there may be a special sense of well-being and closeness between partners, should be discussed. It is also important to mention how some women are able to experience more than one orgasm, possibly several, on the same occasion of love-making, but that the number of orgasms is not usually a measure of the amount of pleasure a woman has received. Similarly, the therapist should emphasize, especially for the benefit of the man, that most women do not appear to feel an overwhelming need to reach orgasm on every occasion of love-making; the experience of high arousal may be sufficiently pleasurable. Some women feel pressurized by their partners to reach orgasm, and this may encourage them to fake orgasm, thus spoiling their enjoyment of sex.

At this point the therapist can introduce the topic of masturbation, by drawing the rapid response cycle which may occur with self-stimulation ((c) in Fig. 2.3). Explaining that many women reach orgasm within two minutes of starting to masturbate can help dispel the notion that a woman always takes longer than a man to become aroused. At the same time the therapist can point out that women often report that orgasm from masturbation is a more intense experience than that from sexual intercourse, although the latter may provide more profound emotional satisfaction. Finally, this is an appropriate time to mention that masturbation by women (and men) is a healthy sexual outlet, and is practised by at least 70-80 per cent of women at some time in their lives.

THE MAN

Sexual anatomy

As when discussing the sexual anatomy of women, it can be helpful to show the couple a picture of a naked man to illustrate natural asymmetry, and differences from the female body form. Then the following should be pointed out in a picture of a man's external genitals: the shaft of the penis, glans penis (emphasizing sensitivity), scrotum and testicles (one testicle usually being higher than the other), and pubic hair (with different distribution to that of a woman—his often extending up to the navel, hers usually having a more emphatic upper border, well below the navel).

The therapist should explain how, just as in women, the appearance of the genitals varies considerably from one man to another. It is important to discuss penis size, and to acknowledge that most men have anxieties about the size of their penis. This may be explained partly by the foreshortening which occurs when a man looks down at his own penis, making it look smaller than that of a man viewed front-on, for example across a changing-room. Many other factors, including dirty jokes, may contribute to the almost universal anxiety that men appear to experience about penis size. It is also worth mentioning Masters and Johnson's finding that there is less variation in size between erect compared with non-erect penises; a penis that is relatively large in the flaccid state usually shows less increase in size than a penis which is smaller when flaccid. Finally, and perhaps most important in this respect, the therapist should explain how penis size is more or less irrelevant to the amount of stimulation a woman receives during sexual intercourse, because sensitivity of the vagina is mostly confined to just inside and around the entrance to the vagina.

For most couples there is little point in discussing a man's internal sexual anatomy as it is fairly complicated, and usually irrelevant to resolution of sexual difficulties. It may be relevant for men with certain problems, such as retrograde ejaculation.

Sexual response

The reader may find it helpful to consult the summary table (Table 2.2) while reading this section.

Again it is useful to employ the graph of sexual response (Fig. 2.7). This serves to emphasize the similarities between the responses of men and women.

Excitement.   The therapist should stress that *erection*, which is equivalent to vaginal lubrication, is a very early response to any form of sexual stimulation and does not mean, as some women believe, that a man must have sexual intercourse very soon in order to avoid discomfort. A very simple explanation of erection might be given, (e.g. extra blood flows into the penis and special valves prevent it flowing out so rapidly). Another point worth making is that during sexual arousal the rigidity or size of an erection may sometimes diminish, but this does not necessarily mean loss of arousal. In addition, the therapist might explain that the *testicles* elevate during this phase, often coming to lie tightly up against the base of the penis.

At this juncture the therapist should point out that for either sex, arousal can easily be disrupted by such factors as anxiety, alcohol, and tiredness.

Plateau.   As in women, this phase is not distinct from the excitement phase. However, one point relevant to a man's response is that anxiety at this stage can cause *either* loss of erection or premature ejaculation. Indeed, these two problems are often closely associated (p. 37).

Orgasm.   The two-stage process involved in ejaculation (emission and expulsion, p. 20) might be mentioned. Orgasm consists of subjective sensations, and contractions of pelvic muscles, especially those around the base of the penis. A man's orgasm is of course distinguished from that of a woman by the occurrence of ejaculation.

With couples in which the man has premature ejaculation, it is important to mention the phenomenon of ejaculatory inevitability ('point of no return'), following which ejaculation cannot be prevented. Some men with premature ejaculation are unaware of this point, and, during treatment, guidance may be provided on how to learn to identify it and to become aware of the sensations that precede it (p. 221).

Resolution.   Apart from indicating that this is a time when the changes that occurred during arousal are reversed, with rapid initial detumescence, followed by slower loss of the remainder of the erection, it is important to discuss the *refractory period*, a phenomenon only found in men. This period after ejaculation, during which a man cannot ejaculate again and is often unable to get a further erection, varies between individuals, and between occasions of love-making, but tends to increase with age from a matter of minutes in a teenager to hours or even days in an older man.

The importance of the resolution phase as a time for closeness and tenderness should again be stressed. It seems that some men cease to attend to their partner once ejaculation has occurred which can cause the partner to feel rejected.

THE EFFECTS OF AGEING

The therapist should briefly mention the effects of ageing on the sexuality of women and men (p. 22 and p. 16). This may not be relevant to a couple in their teens or twenties, but should certainly be covered in couples who are older than that. The therapist should highlight the positive effects of ageing as well as those that appear to suggest a decline in performance and enjoyment. When discussing the changes with age in women the therapist should emphasize that the ability to enjoy sexuality is usually maintained long after the menopause and that help can be provided for some of the negative effects of the menopause. For example, reduced vaginal lubrication will usually be improved by hormone cream. An older man may require more sexual stimulation in order to have and maintain his erection; he may also need more stimulation to reach orgasm. However, with ageing, the need to ejaculate often declines, a man tends to develop more control over his speed of ejaculation, and he should be more able to provide pleasure to his partner through his greater experience. For both sexes, continuation of sexual activity appears to be one of the best ways of averting the negative sexual affects of ageing.

When the therapist has completed this account, the couple should be encouraged to ask questions. The therapist should also reassure them that questions of a factual nature are welcome at any time during therapy.

CONCLUSIONS

The educational component of sex therapy can be extremely valuable. Indeed, in helping some couples this is the most important aspect of therapy. Although education about sexuality will occur as an on-going process during the therapeutic programme, it is strongly recommended that the therapist devotes some time to the provision of information about male and female sexual anatomy and response. This should be backed up by recommending suitable reading material. It is unwise to assume that a couple have a sophisticated knowledge of sexuality; very often a couple who give this impression will be unwilling to admit to areas of ignorance, or be unaware of their blindspots. A fairly didactic educational session, in which pictures are used, is helpful. This session should be tailored to the needs and problems, as well as the educational level, of the individual couple. Finally, in order to provide information in an accurate and confident fashion, the therapist must have a sound knowledge of human sexual anatomy and response before embarking on sex therapy.

11

Helping with general relationship problems

Problems in the general relationship are often apparent at the outset of sex therapy with couples, and in other cases they may come to the fore as therapy proceeds. A couple may describe their difficulty in global terms, such as not getting on, continually arguing about nothing, and never agreeing about things. However, specific complaints can usually be elicited, and include, for example, complaints by one or both partners that insufficient affection is shown, disagreements about social outings or use of leisure time, one partner's resentment about the role of the other partner, or lack of appreciation of the other's role, and disagreements over policies concerning discipline of children. Sex therapy can often continue in spite of such issues. However, they must be addressed if they impede progress in the sexual relationship. In this chapter we shall briefly consider some approaches that have proved effective in the management of general relationship issues within the context of a sex therapy programme. The reader who wishes to gain a more thorough understanding of general relationship therapy is referred elsewhere (e.g. Stuart 1980).

The approach described here is based on similar principles to sex therapy, including identification of target problems, agreeing on tasks which provide a means of gradually overcoming the problem, and exploring any difficulties that are encountered by the couple to further clarify the nature of the problems in their relationship. In general, this relatively directive approach appears

to be superior to other approaches, such as those of a more inter-
pretive kind (Crowe 1978).

Once it becomes apparent that there are difficulties in a couple's
general relationship which must be addressed, the couple should
be given a simple rationale for this approach. It could, for example,
be pointed out that the generally tense atmosphere between them
is partly a result of specific problems. Solutions to such problems
will be more straightforward than attempting to deal with the
tense atmosphere itself. In addition to improvements in the problems tackled during therapy, the couple may go on to deal with
other problems in similar ways. Changes in the partner's attitudes
to each other may also allow them to re-evaluate other aspects of
their relationship, so that improvements in specific areas may
generalize to the relationship as a whole.

Assessment

If it is obvious that there are significant problems in a couple's
general relationship, the next stage in assessing them is to determine whether these difficulties can be tackled briefly while the
couple remain in sex therapy, or whether the issues are paramount and therefore require intensive marital therapy. It is
inadvisable to attempt to carry out concurrent programmes of
sex and marital therapy with the same couple because this usually
causes unhelpful confusion for the couple. It is sometimes found
that the general relationship is so disturbed that any form of
therapy stands little chance of success. This is likely to be the
case if one partner clearly lacks any feelings of affection for the
other.

The first stage in tackling general relationship issues consists,
as in sex therapy, of a detailed assessment of the couple's problems. The therapist should aim to move the partners away from
general criticisms of the relationship and each other to more
specific complaints which allow a greater possibility of change.
The couple are prompted to consider what sort of relationship
they wish to develop or return to, rather than to simply focus on
what they dislike. In particular the therapist should try to help
the partners answer the following questions:

1. What are their complaints (i.e. what is the problem according to each partner)?

2. What behaviour does each partner wish the other to change?
3. Under what circumstances does this need to occur?
4. What will be the consequences for each partner of such changes?

The following are examples of such assessments:

A couple in which the wife had lost interest in sex were making slow progress during sex therapy because the woman was rarely in the mood even to begin sessions of sensate focus. Careful analysis revealed that her husband spent considerable time in the evenings talking to her about things which happened at work. However, he rarely asked her how she had got on at home, especially in managing their two young children. When the wife broached the subject of her day her husband appeared to lose interest and usually found an excuse to do something else, such as reading the newspaper. He said he thought his wife ought to be more interested in his work, but admitted that he neglected to show the same regard for her equally busy domestic commitments. When asked to specify more precisely what type of changes they each wanted, the wife explained that she did not want to spend hours talking about her day, but would be glad of the chance to let off steam and to feel that she had her husband's support. She agreed that she was interested in what happened to her husband at work, but said she would find it easier to show her interest if he also paid heed to her. In addition, she thought it likely that if their relationship could change in this way she would feel more enthusiastic about beginning the homework assignments in the sex therapy programme.

A couple who entered treatment because of the husband's premature ejaculation had only had two sessions of sensate focus during the first three weeks of the programme. When the therapist explored the reasons for this the wife complained that her husband was affectionate only when he wanted to have sex. The husband had not been aware of this, and added that his wife often did not let him know how she was feeling, but allowed her resentment to build up until eventually they had a row. When the wife was asked to be more specific in terms of how and when she would like her husband to show her affection, she said she wanted him occasionally to put an arm round her or hold hands when they were out walking, or when at the pub. She thought this would help her feel that her husband was fond of her, rather than any demonstration of affection by him always being a prelude to sex. For his part, the husband said that he would rather his wife told him immediately when bad feelings began to develop. Both agreed that this would probably reduce the frequency and intensity of their rows.

Target behaviours may not be easily identified. A useful technique, which can be therapeutic in its own right, is to ask the partners to think about those aspects of each other's behaviour which they like, and those which they dislike. The partners should independently write down these points before the next treatment session. In addition, they should note down changes which they would like to see in the partner's behaviour, particularly *positive* desired changes (e.g. 'taking me out socially more often') rather than *negative* ones (e.g. 'not nagging me so much'). This is discussed further below (p. 188). Finally, they should also record aspects of the partner's behaviour which is particularly pleasing. The partners should bring their lists to the next session without having discussed them in the meantime.

In the session they are asked to read their lists to each other. The therapist will often need to assist the partners to be more specific in their points (e.g. 'showing more affection' might be clarified further, such as 'giving me a kiss in the morning, putting an arm round me when watching T.V.'). This usually provides a useful basis for establishing what changes should be the focus for therapy. Indicating their likes as well as their dislikes helps provide a more rational assessment of the relationship.

Strategies

Once *target behaviours* and *goals* can be identified clearly in this way, there are various means of helping a couple to make the desired changes in their relationship. First, the partners should be asked what they think each might do to improve the situation. This encourages them to take responsibility for their relationship. However, most couples need further advice from the therapist. Possible suggestions are discussed below.

The principles inherent in this relatively directive approach to general relationship issues are essentially the same as those involved in sex therapy. In other words, the therapist encourages the partners to agree on tasks they will endeavour to carry out before the next session. At that session their progress is reviewed. If they have been successful they are encouraged to continue with the approach, and, if possible, to extend it further. If they have been unsuccessful, the therapist helps them analyse in detail what happened and why. It may become apparent that the task was too demanding and that a simpler task would be more appropriate, or that another approach must be tried, or that the target problem must be reassessed in case it is secondary to other and perhaps more fundamental issues.

The following are the particular strategies which have been found useful in the management of general relationship problems in the context of sex therapy.

1. *Detailed monitoring.* The partners can be asked to keep detailed but specific notes about the target problems. This can be helpful in its own right, as it is known that record-keeping of this kind often reduces the intensity or frequency of occurrence of a wide range of problems (Rimm and Masters 1979). It may lead to a re-evaluation of the problem, when, for example, it is found that it occurs very infrequently. It may also produce a new picture of the problem, with simple solutions being obvious.

One couple, for example, both complained that the wife's irritability with her two sons produced an unpleasant atmosphere in the home. Detailed record-keeping by both partners suggested that incidents early in the day coloured the interactions for the rest of the day. The husband suggested that the wife should stay in bed until the boys, who were at their most boisterous in the morning, were ready for school. This simple step both reduced the wife's nagging, and also allowed her to feel that she was a more successful mother because she was warmer generally with the boys.

2. *Specific suggestions.* Very often specific suggestions to a couple are sufficient, at least as an initial step.

For example, a couple who complained that their life had become very humdrum since their children were born were advised to book a babysitter once a week on a regular basis as a way of ensuring that they went out together at least weekly. When the couple raised the objection that on some such nights there would be nothing special to do, the therapist suggested that the most important need was for them to have time together away from the home environment. They then agreed that on some nights they would go to the cinema, on others to their local pub, and on others to one of their nearby eating places.

This may appear naively simple. However, it is surprising how often couples are encouraged by a third party making specific suggestions, enabling them to break out of a chronic pattern with which they have long been dissatisfied.

3. *Contracting*. This is one of the most useful strategies in helping with general relationship problems. In essence it consists of both partners trying to alter their behaviour, on a mutually agreed basis. There are several very important ways in which the effectiveness of this strategy can be improved:

(i) The changes which are intended must be very *specific*. For example, 'doing more around the house' is not a suitable goal, but might be broken down into specific behaviours such as 'washing-up the dishes three times a week', 'tidying the study once a week', or 'finishing a painting job'.

(ii) The contract should be based on *positive requests*. Thus it should not include requests to reduce the frequency of behaviour (e.g. nagging, going to the pub, coming home late from work) but only to introduce new behaviour or to increase the frequency of behaviour which already occurs.

(iii) The intended changes should be relatively *independent*, not reciprocal. Thus contracts ought not to consist of arrangements such as, 'If I do . . . , you should do . . . in exchange'. Although the principal aim of contracting is to assist both partners to change their behaviour in a way which is to the liking of the other, direct linking of target behaviours in this way is akin to coercion and provides too much opportunity for failure. The alternative approach, in which partners try to introduce a series of independent changes, allows for partial improvement (which is often a realistic outcome, at least in the short-term).

(iv) The targets should be *specified by the partners*, not by the therapist. The therapist's role is to assist the partners to draw up their contracts, but not specify the precise details.

Once the contract is agreed it should be recorded in writing by the therapist, and each partner given a copy. The couple are then asked to try before the next session to introduce as many of the changes as possible. Some couples find it helpful if they keep a written record, but it is best if each partner only records the frequency of his or her own behaviours, not those of the partner.

At the next session the therapist helps the couple to examine their progress, exploring the reasons for any difficulties that have occurred. It may become apparent that the nature of the contract must be changed.

Examples of such contracts are provided in Table 11.1 in order to clarify this procedure for the reader.

TABLE 11.1

Examples of marital contracts

1

Peter would like Jane to:	*Jane would like Peter to:*
Have supper ready by 7.00p.m. most nights.	Take her out socially at least once a fortnight.
Encourage him to spend a few hours each weekend in a sporting pursuit (e.g. squash, running, swimming), and to join him in this whenever possible.	Show her more affection at times other than before sex, by kissing her in the morning, putting an arm round her sometimes when watching TV, and occasionally holding her hand when out in public.
Prepare a special meal for them both once a fortnight.	Offer to take out their children on his own once each weekend (e.g. to local park, sporting event, or shopping).
Suggest things they might do socially, rather than always leaving him to decide.	Come to bed by 11.00p.m.

2

Vivian would like Mark to:	*Mark would like Vivian to:*
Share with her the painting of their kitchen.	Begin to lose ½ stone in weight.
Spend part of each weekend looking clean and tidy (instead of always looking scruffy).	Encourage him to invite some of their friends for a meal.
Arrange to be at home on a particular evening each week to look after the children when she wishes to attend an aerobics class and afterwards have a drink with her friends.	Kiss him when they get home from work *before* they begin to tell each other how difficult the day has been.

4. *Use of the personal pronoun.* As was noted earlier when sensate focus was described (p. 132), a very helpful strategy is to suggest that each partner begins as many statements as possible with the personal pronoun 'I'. Thus a statement such as 'you make me so angry' could be replaced by 'I feel so angry when

you . . . ', and one such as 'we could go to the cinema' could be replaced by 'I want to go to the cinema'. This can help improve communication between partners, and also encourages each partner to take responsibility for his or her own feelings and inclinations.

5. *Communication periods.* When a couple complain that they never discuss things, or that any attempt to do so ends in a row, the therapist might suggest that they allocate specific periods for free discussion. For example, a couple could agree that three times a week they will put aside a half-hour period during which they will freely discuss whether they wish, including, for example, the day's events, reasons for discontent, and things they have enjoyed. This arrangement works best if the partners agree that they will not argue during this period, however they are feeling. This may enable them to express frustrations or other negative feelings without fear of immediate strife. In addition, the partners should be encouraged to use the personal pronoun, as described above.

When a couple anticipate that this will be too difficult, they might be encouraged to begin by discussing in the treatment sessions some topic of disagreement. The therapist can then help them to do this, as suggested above, in a constructive and non-hostile fashion, using the personal pronoun.

6. *Special events.* A useful suggestion for some couples, especially those who complain that their relationship is monotonous, is that occasionally each of the partners should devote themselves to organizing a day, or an evening, in a way that the partner will enjoy. For example, one husband said he would plan pleasant surprises for his wife (e.g. a special meal, a film, the theatre). A woman said she would prepare a special meal for her husband, including food and wine that she knew he particularly enjoyed.

CONCLUSIONS

We have already noted how important it is when assessing the suitability of couples for sex therapy to identify those who have major problems in their general relationship. Such couples are usually best considered for marital rather than sex therapy. However, some couples are accepted for sex therapy in spite of general relationship difficulties because it is not thought that these preclude a successful outcome. In addition, previously unrecognized general relationship issues quite often come to the fore during sex therapy. In such cases it is often possible to offer help using some of the suggestions in this chapter. They have the advantage of being based on similar principles to the sex therapy programme, and therefore can be incorporated into treatment fairly easily. They are also useful in the management of couples who present with marital rather than sexual problems, provided both partners show sufficient motivation.

12

The end of treatment

Earlier in this book we discussed how the sex therapy programme should be introduced in a careful and structured fashion. Similar care must be paid to ending treatment. In this chapter we will consider how the therapist should plan the end of treatment, the different reasons why treatment ends, and how progress can be systematically assessed.

PLANNING THE END OF TREATMENT

The therapist should prepare a couple for termination of treatment from the outset. Thus they should be told roughly how long treatment is likely to last and what number of treatment sessions might be involved. Although sex therapy is generally much briefer than some forms of psychological treatment, such as intensive psychotherapy, the programme nevertheless involves a substantial time commitment for both couples and therapist. A couple should not begin with unreasonable expectations about the length of treatment. However, the therapist should also explain that there is not an absolutely rigid time schedule, and that the duration of treatment will depend on their progress.

If after several weeks of weekly therapy sessions a couple's difficulties are beginning to resolve, it may be appropriate to extend the gap between treatment sessions to two weeks. However, the therapist must exercise care in doing this. Failures during a less frequent schedule of sessions are often more difficult to resolve, especially if they occur shortly after a treatment session, because they may be repeated and cause a couple to feel demoralized before the next session.

When treatment is clearly coming to an end a useful strategy is to suggest a three or four week gap between the penultimate and final treatment sessions. This provides time for consolidation of progress, while the couple still feel supported by the therapist. It also allows the couple to gradually regain their sense of independence and autonomy (p. 154).

During the final treatment sessions the couple should be prepared for possible future problems. After explaining that it is not uncommon for difficulties to recur, the therapist should examine with the couple what they will do if this happens. A sensible approach is to recommend that they re-implement the sex therapy programme, or at least some aspects of it, including non-genital and genital sensate focus. This is often sufficient to resolve further problems without outside help.

It is also helpful to offer couples a three months follow-up appointment. Again this helps maintain a sense of support from the therapist. In this session the therapist can review any difficulties that have occurred, and how the couple dealt with them. It also provides the therapist with a chance to assess the effectiveness of treatment.

REASONS FOR TREATMENT ENDING

There are several reasons why a sex therapy programme with a couple might end, and these are considered below.

Entirely successful outcome

Naturally the best outcome of sex therapy is one where the presenting difficulty has been resolved, and the couple are now entirely satisfied with their relationship. The therapist usually should avoid tackling further problems beyond those which at the outset were agreed as being the focus of treatment. Some inexperienced therapists tend to be over-enthusiastic and, inappropriately, try to improve every aspect of a couple's sexual relationship. This can be self-defeating because, first, it may mean that failure results, perhaps spoiling the success obtained with the original problem. Secondly, the couple may develop the unrealistic expectation that a perfect sexual relationship is the only acceptable goal of treatment. Thirdly, it represents inefficient use of a therapist's time, which would be better used for the treatment of other couples with more severe difficulties. Residual difficulties will sometimes resolve unaided, or with brief advice from the therapist, because the partners are now more confident about their sexual relationship and more able to discuss sexual matters. An example of this concerned a very young couple who entered treatment because of the man's erectile dysfunction. This resolved fairly quickly. It then became apparent that his partner never experienced orgasm with him, although she was easily orgasmic through masturbation on her own. The therapist's supervisor advised against further treatment for this problem because the couple were now well-informed, were developing a varied and rewarding sexual relationship, and the woman was happy to show her partner how to provide her with more effective genital stimulation. As predicted, by the time of the three month follow-up she was orgasmic with her partner, during both foreplay and sexual intercourse.

Partial success
Often sex therapy is only partly successful. Most couples are happy to accept this—a fact which therapists must recognize in order to avoid prolonging therapy unnecessarily.

Partial success sometimes means that the presenting problem is only present intermittently. In other cases it may be that the problem itself has not changed but that the couple have been able to accept it. A third possibility is that the problem still occurs but less intensely. For example, one couple entered treatment because the man experienced severe premature ejaculation, and by the end of treatment he had gained good ejaculatory control on most occasions of sexual intercourse. However, rapid ejaculation still sometimes occurred, usually when the man was tired, or when sexual intercourse was resumed after his partner had ceased menstruating. This couple's outcome was recorded as 'presenting problem largely resolved, although some difficulties still experienced'. The couple happily accepted this pattern of sexual activity, and were not unduly perturbed by the occasional episode of rapid ejaculation.

Termination of unsuccessful treatment by the therapist

Sex therapy will sometimes be terminated by the therapist even though treatment has not been successful. There are three reasons why this happens. First, it may become apparent that a couple will not benefit from further treatment. Once this happens it is unwise to prolong treatment further because of possible demoralization for both the couple and the therapist, and because it represents inefficient use of therapeutic time. If no substantial progress has occurred within ten sessions of treatment, it is usually pointless continuing. Termination need not be abrupt, however, but can take place over two or three treatment sessions during which the therapist should allow the couple to avoid demoralization as far as possible by encouraging them to focus on whatever gains have occurred, however small these might be. It also allows the therapist to consider what further help, if any, might be needed.

A second reason for a therapist terminating treatment is because it has become obvious that another approach is indicated. The most common examples are: (i) when major general relationship difficulties, not identified at the outset, become apparent—either a change in therapeutic approach, or referral for marital therapy, may then be necessary; and (ii) when it appears that one of the partners requires individual help, perhaps for a psychiatric disorder, or because an individual approach to the sexual problem now seems more appropriate (p. 216).

The third reason for a therapist terminating treatment, and one to which therapists should always be alert, is that the treatment programme appears increasingly likely to confront a couple with the fragility of their relationship, maybe even that the relationship is sustained by the sexual dysfunction. The author does not believe it to be the business of a therapist to force such confrontation on a couple if it is apparent this might precipitate the break-up of the relationship. Instead, the couple should be allowed gradually to withdraw from treatment, again being allowed the opportunity to save face by attributing whatever benefits they wish to the treatment, however unrealistic this might be. For example, a couple in late middle-age entered treatment because of the wife's very longstanding problem of primary vaginismus. Following fairly lengthy treatment, in which the couple reported being more able to caress and arouse each other, no progress was made with regard to the presenting problem. However, the couple's relationship appeared to be sustained in part by their expectation that consummation would one day occur. The therapist realized that resolution of the wife's vaginismus was unlikely because of her very entrenched fears of sexual commitment, and therefore ended treatment. The couple expressed considerable satisfaction with their progress, in spite of there having been no change in their main problem.

Termination of treatment by the couple

Treatment sometimes ends because a couple indicate that they do not wish to continue, or because, without warning, they fail to attend any further treatment sessions. There are three common reasons for this. First, either the couple, or one of the partners, might have found the treatment programme unacceptable, or think that it will not help. Secondly, the couple may have been unsuccessful in their attempts to carry out their latest homework assignments and feel too embarrassed or demoralized to attend further sessions. This situation emphasizes the need to ensure that couples realize at the outset of therapy that difficult patches are to be expected, and may even be essential before they can develop a fuller understanding of their problems. Thirdly, a couple sometimes reach a stage when they think that their sexual relationship has improved sufficiently, and do not wish to pursue the treatment programme further.

In any of these situations, the therapist usually ought to telephone or write to the couple to determine what has happened and to offer a further appointment if indicated. A couple who have encountered difficulties will sometimes be relieved to discover that their therapist not only appears unperturbed by their being unable to carry out their homework assignments, but, on the contrary, encourages them to see this as an opportunity to develop a fuller understanding of their problem.

The couple's relationship ends

Sex therapy can be confronting for a couple whose relationship is fragile. Occasionally a couple will end their relationship during treatment. One partner may have entered treatment hoping it will fail, so that the relationship could be ended justifiably, all possible steps having been taken to resolve the couple's difficulties. A relationship sometimes ends because one partner has an affair; a very rare consequence of sex therapy is that one partner experiences greater freedom to establish sexual relationships because his or her sexual problem has resolved.

Even when a couple's relationship ends it is sometimes possible to continue providing treatment for one partner. For example, two unmarried students entered treatment because the girl had severe vaginismus, but ended this relationship after eight treatment sessions. The girl, however, continues in individual therapy aimed at helping her gain more confidence so that she would feel more able to have sexual intercourse in a subsequent relationship should she wish to do so.

In a consecutive series of 100 couples who entered sex therapy in our clinic, 70 completed treatment, 20 dropped out, and in 10 cases treatment was terminated by the therapist. Couples who completed treatment had a mean of 14 treatment sessions (including the initial assessment), with a range from 7 to 37 sessions. However, rarely did treatment continue for more than 20 sessions. The actual results of treatment, and the factors which are associated with outcome, are discussed in the next chapter.

ASSESSMENT OF OUTCOME

Therapists are advised to monitor the progress of couples who enter therapy. This can provide valuable feedback on how effective their treatment is and help prevent them from developing either an exaggerated or unduly pessimistic opinion of their effectiveness.

Outcome can be monitored by obtaining simple ratings at the end of treatment, and at any subsequent follow-up interviews. Preferably, ratings should also be obtained before treatment begins. These can be made by the therapist and also by the couple. Ideally, three types of ratings should be made; one concerning *changes in the presenting problem,* a second which reflects the couple's current *satisfaction with their sexual relationship,* and

a third concerning the couple's *general relationship*. In rating changes in the presenting problem the following scale has been found useful:
(1) presenting problem resolved;
(2) presenting problem largely resolved, although some difficulty still experienced;
(3) some improvement, but presenting problem largely unresolved;
(4) no change;
(5) problem worse.

A similar scale might be used to record the couple's satisfaction with their sexual relationship:
(1) completely satisfied with the sexual relationship;
(2) largely satisfied with the sexual relationship, but some dissatisfaction;
(3) some satisfaction with the sexual relationship, but largely dissatisfied;
(4) complete dissatisfaction with the sexual relationship.

By changing the word 'sexual' to 'general' this scale could also be used to record the couple's satisfaction with their general relationship. All of these scales may be open to bias, especially if rated only by the therapist. However, they do encourage the therapist to think critically about the outcome of treatment.

For the therapist who wishes to extend the evaluation of therapy further, there are many possibilities. For example, standardized questionnaires might be used to obtain pre-treatment, post-treatment, and follow-up assessments, and then examined for changes. The Maudsley Marital Questionnaire is one instrument suitable for this purpose (Crowe 1978). It includes ratings of sexual, general, and social aspects of a relationship (and adjustment at work), all made on 10-point scales, and can be completed by each partner in a few minutes. A more lengthy and probing assessment of sexual function is provided by the Sexual Interaction Inventory (LoPiccolo and Steger 1974).

A simple questionnaire for assessing pleasant and unpleasant feelings in five typical sexual situations, which was introduced in a study by Carney *et al.* (1978), has proved to be a sensitive measure of change. However, it should be noted that anomalous results are sometimes obtained for ratings by men of unpleasant feelings, especially pre-treatment, when many men appear unwilling to admit to such feelings. They are sometimes more willing to do so at the end of treatment.

CONCLUSIONS

The ending of treatment should receive as much care and planning as its initiation. Termination should be anticipated well in advance, and should be gradual rather than abrupt. Therapists are advised to provide at least one follow-up session some months after treatment has ended. Treatment may be terminated by the couple. There are several possible reasons for this; the therapist should be particularly on guard for couples who leave treatment because they are embarrassed about their poor progress. Every effort should be made to re-engage such couples in treatment.

Therapists are urged to try to assess the outcome of their couples in a standardized fashion. Simple ratings can be used for this purpose. This is helpful because it emphasizes that outcome of treatment is often a partial success, rather than either absolute success or failure. Fortunately, many couples are happy to accept such an outcome.

13

Research findings concerning sex therapy with couples

Since the introduction of the current approaches to sexual problems, clinical enthusiasm has tended to be far ahead of research
efforts in this field. It is now apparent that the enormous optimism
which initially greeted the appearance of sex therapy at the
beginning of the 1970s was only partly justified. Fortunately,
sufficient research has been conducted for clinical practice to be
based on a more substantial footing. Some of the research findings which are important with regard to the provision of sex
therapy for couples will be reviewed in this chapter. First,
reports concerning the effectiveness of sex therapy will be considered, including the long-term outcome, and factors which
appear to be important in the prediction of outcome. Secondly,
studies comparing the effectiveness of sex therapy with other
methods of treatment will be discussed. Thirdly, studies will be
reviewed in which three important components in the application of sex therapy have been evaluated, namely single therapists
and co-therapists, the frequency of treatment sessions, and the
use of self-help treatments.

THE OUTCOME OF SEX THERAPY

Short-term outcome

The original outcome stastistics published by Masters and Johnson
(1970) were remarkable. These workers adopted the unusual

approach of only reporting treatment failures. Although other people naturally assumed that all those couples who were not treatment failures had a successful outcome, this appears to have been an unwarranted assumption according to a more recent publication by Masters and Johnson (1979, p. 381).

In addition, their outcome statistics are probably open to other criticisms, including the uncertain nature of the outcome criteria (Zilbergeld and Evans 1980) and, as they themselves have admitted, biases in patient selection (Masters and Johnson 1970). However, their statistics are a natural starting point for discussion, as they were the major reason why sex therapy received such an enthusiastic welcome. Their failure rates for the various dysfunctions at the end of treatment were, in summary, as follows (using their terminology):

Orgasmic dysfunction	
primary	16.6 per cent
situational	22.8 per cent
Vaginismus	nil failures
Impotence	
primary	40.6 per cent
secondary	26.3 per cent
Premature ejaculation	2.2 per cent
Ejaculatory incompetence	17.6 per cent

The reader will note that, at the time of reporting these figures, Masters and Johnson did not distinguish problems concerning sexual interest or desire. Their overall failure rate, based on the treatment of more than 500 couples and individuals without partners, was 18.9 per cent. In a five-year follow-up of 313 couples (all post-treatment non-failures) they found an overall relapse rate of only 5.1 per cent. Relapses were more common in couples who had presented with secondary impotence (11.1 per cent).

The outcome statistics reported by other workers have been far more modest than those of Masters and Johnson. In Oxford, for example, Bancroft and Coles (1976) reviewed therapists' retrospective ratings of outcome for 78 couples who entered sex therapy. A 'successful outcome' was recorded in 37 per cent, 'worthwhile improvement' in 31 per cent, and 'no worthwhile improvement' or 'dropped out' in 32 per cent. These results were similar to those being reported elsewhere in the United Kingdom at about the same time (Duddle 1975; Milne 1976).

More recent data is available from the Oxford clinic (Hawton 1982). For 100 couples who entered treatment, at termination the presenting problem was rated as resolved or largely resolved in 66 per cent, largely unresolved but with some improvement in 12 per cent, unchanged in 21 per cent, and worse in 1 per cent. The best outcome was obtained with vaginismus (presenting problem resolved or largely resolved in 79 per cent of cases), and erectile dysfunction (81 per cent). At the three month follow-up interviews the post-treatment gains appeared to have persisted in most couples who attended, although it was not possible to reassess 24 per cent of the couples.

So far only uncontrolled studies have been considered. Studies in which sex therapy has been compared with other forms of treatment are discussed later (p. 207). However, Heiman and LoPiccolo (1983) compared changes in the sexual and general adjustment of couples who received treatment for a variety of sexual problems with those changes which occurred while they were on a one to two-month waiting-list. Only slight changes were found while on the waiting-list, but there were significant improvements in most aspects of the couples' sexual functioning and general relationships following treatment. There are, however, serious problems with using waiting-list controls, including the likelihood that couples temporarily suspend efforts at improving their relationships while awaiting treatment.

Long-term outcome

Very little information is available concerning the long-term outcome following sex therapy. The five-year follow-up carried out by Masters and Johnson (1970) has already been noted. One of the main problems encountered by other people who have conducted long-term follow-up studies after sex therapy is the large number of couples for whom it has not been possible to arrange follow-up interviews. Two further important issues are, first, the question of how to interpret findings for couples who have separated, especially if one or both partners have established further, non-dysfunctional relationships, and secondly, how to attribute sexual adjustment at follow-up to sex therapy rather than to independent events.

In a study in which sex therapy (provided either by individual therapists or by co-therapists) was compared with marital therapy and relaxation, in the treatment of couples with sexual dysfunction, Crowe *et al.* (1981) found good maintenance of therapeutic gains one year after the end of treatment. A quarter of the couples were unavailable for follow-up; a few of these (8.3 per cent of the total sample) had separated.

Heiman and LoPiccolo (1983) also conducted one year follow-up interviews with couples who had entered a treatment study in which daily and weekly treatment sessions were compared. Again, relatively good maintenance of therapeutic gains was found at the one-year follow-up, although the authors commented that 'couples tend to let sex become a routine, low-priority activity after therapy ends. Thus, while specific symptoms did not recur, indication of the quality of the total sexual experience showed a decline'. However, their findings are marred by a 69 per cent loss of couples at the one-year follow-up.

In Holland, Dekker and Everaerd (1983) attempted to follow up by postal questionnaire 140 couples who had received treatment for sexual dysfunction between five and eight years previously. Although 63 per cent of the couples responded to the follow-up enquiry, only 46 per cent of the total returned usable questionnaires. This study also suffered from inclusion of retrospective ratings of pre- and immediate post-treatment adjustment, although these measures were shown to correlate significantly with more complicated measures used at the time of treatment. Most of the positive changes which had occurred in both sexual and non-sexual interaction between the partners during treatment were sustained throughout the follow-up period. Of 112 couples for whom the information was available, 21 per cent had divorced by the time of the follow-up. Divorced partners had before treatment shown greater 'dissatisfaction with coitus' than other partners.

Watson and Brockman (1982) investigated the outcome of 116 couples who entered sex therapy in a clinic at a London teaching hospital between 3 and 24 months (mean 13.3 months) earlier. They were only able to interview 53 per cent of the couples. Follow-up rates did not differ, however, between those couples who had benefited from treatment and those who had done badly. Watson and Brockman reported that, 'at most', 55 per cent of the successfully treated couples had maintained their improvement, but the rest had relapsed, almost a quarter of these having separated. Of nine unsuccessfully treated couples, eight had separated or divorced, and one reported improved 'marital accord'. Of 24 couples for whom sex therapy had been thought inadvisable or impracticable, 11 had separated or divorced. Sexual adjustment had not improved in any of these 24 couples. The authors concluded that a reasonably satisfactory treatment outcome was found at follow-up in perhaps about two-fifths of those treated. The overall separation of divorce rate was 35.5 per cent. It was much lower among couples who had a successful end-of-treatment outcome than in those who had a poor outcome or for whom treatment was contraindicated. It seems likely that the clinic on which this study was based probably accepted for treatment many more couples with general marital problems than might be the case elsewhere.

Finally, Levine and Agle (1978) reported that couples who were followed up one year after having sex therapy because of erectile dysfunction showed very poor maintenance of the original benefits of treatment.

Although some studies have suggested that the results of treatment remain fairly stable after treament ends, at least in the short term, others have suggested poorer longer-term outcome. One suspects that there will be considerable differences between the long-term outcome for different types of dysfunction. For example, it might reasonably be predicted that once vaginismus has resolved this will usually be permanent, partly because of the phobic nature of the problem and partly because of the otherwise good sexual adjustment of many women with this problem when they first present for help. It also seems likely that erectile dysfunction will show greater recurrence because of the vulnerability of the erectile response to stress, and the possible contribution of physical factors in some cases. One would expect that many couples treated for impaired sexual interest would have further problems because interpersonal difficulties would often have been important in causing the problem in the first place, and would quite commonly recur.

The rate of separation in couples whose treatment is unsuccessful is relatively high. This probably reflects the severity of disturbance in the relationship of these couples when entering treatment, rather than a failure of treatment *per se.* There is an obvious need for further prospective long-term outcome studies, preferably involving standardized assessment procedures. Information is particularly required concerning the long-term outcome for the various types of sexual dysfunctions.

Factors associated with outcome

It is often difficult to predict a couple's response to sex therapy. As noted earlier in this chapter, the nature of the presenting problem is one important factor. Vaginismus and premature ejaculation generally have a good outcome, success occurs a little less frequently with erectile dysfunction, and relatively poor outcome is not unusual when the presenting problem is impaired sexual interest. The presenting problem is, however, only one factor associated with outcome; other characteristics of couples are also likely to be important.

It is unfortunate that there has been little prospective research of such prognostic factors. There are, however, some findings based on retrospective examination of case material and clinical impressions that have emerged during the course of treatment. The following factors are those which at present appear to have important associations with outcome:

1. *Quality of the general relationship.* Not surprisingly, the degree of general harmony between partners has emerged in several studies as the most important factor influencing outcome (Fordney-Settlage 1975; O'Connor 1976; Stoll 1978; Whitehead and Mathews 1981; Snyder and Berg 1983), with the extent of commitment to the relationship being an important aspect of this (Stoll 1978). The unpublished results of a recent prospective study support these findings and also suggest that women tend to rate their relationships more accurately than do men (Hawton 1983).

2. *Psychopathology.* O'Connor (1976) reported that if either partner has a psychiatric disorder this tends to be associated with poor outcome. However, a prospective study, in which standard measures of psychopathology as well as clinical ratings were obtained, failed to support this finding (Hawton 1983). Presumably, whether psychopathology emerges as a factor will depend on the extent to which people with psychiatric disorders are

accepted for, or excluded from sex therapy in the first place (p. 99).

3. *Motivation.* Treatment outcome is bound to be related in part to the motivation of a couple (Cooper 1969). An interesting observation by Fordney-Settlage (1975) was that outcome was particularly determined by the male partner's motivation. This observation has been supported by preliminary findings from a prospective study (Hawton 1983). One possible explanation is that the model of sexuality embodied in sex therapy is more acceptable to women than to men, and therefore the result of therapy with a couple will depend on the extent to which the man is enthusiastic about solving the problem, even if this means approaching sexual interaction in a way that is not customary for him. This suggestion clearly warrants further investigation, with attention being paid to whether there may be differences with regard to the nature of the presenting problem.

4. *Duration of the sexual problem.* Several authors have reported that the outcome of sex therapy may be poorer the longer the duration of the presenting problem (Cooper 1969, 1970; O'Connor 1976).

5. *Previous sexual adjustment.* Outcome may also depend on the extent to which partners have previously been sexually responsive (Cooper 1969) or derived pleasure from their sexual relationship (Whitehead and Mathews 1981). Furthermore, the more disturbed a couple's sexual relationship at the outset of therapy, the more difficult it may be to help them (Hawton 1983). Only two studies have addressed the question of the extent to which partners find each other sexually attractive at the outset of therapy, and in both of these it was found that greater attraction between partners heralded a better outcome (Whitehead and Mathews 1977, 1981).

6. *Early progress in therapy.* The extent to which couples make progress early in treatment (Stoll 1978), and similarly the extent to which they engage in the sensate focus exercises during the first three treatment sessions (Hawton 1983), are a very good indication of the likely eventual outcome.

Although this summary of the studies of factors associated with the outcome of sex therapy reveals some interesting findings, the situation is not entirely clear because there may be important interactions between the factors. For example, motivation and early progress in therapy are likely to be related, but they might in turn reflect a more fundamental factor, such as the quality of the general relationship between partners.

SEX THERAPY COMPARED WITH OTHER METHODS OF TREATMENT

In this section, controlled studies in which sex therapy has been compared with other forms of treatment will be briefly reviewed. The studies will be considered in chronological order. No reference will be made to studies comparing other forms of treatment (e.g. systematic desensitization versus drug-assisted treatments); for a review of these the reader should consult Wright *et al.* (1977).

A somewhat unusual evaluation of sex therapy was provided by Kockott *et al.* (1975). After finding that most couples in which the men had erectile dysfunction failed to improve with systematic desensitization, four sessions of 'routine medical treatment', or being placed on a waiting-list, they then provided 12 of the couples with sex therapy using a modified Masters and Johnson approach. Of these, eight were reported to be either 'cured' or 'improved'. Although not a proper controlled study (a cumulative effective of different therapies being one possible explanation for the result), the authors suggested that it provided evidence that sex therapy was superior to the other approaches.

Ansari (1976) also studied treatment of men with erectile dysfunction. He compared three forms of treatment: (i) modified Masters and Johnson therapy; (ii) chemotherapy (a tranquillizer); and (iii) non-specific treatment. At the end of the treatment period and at an eight-month follow-up, neither of the active forms of treatment appeared to have been more effective than the non-specific treatment. Although this study appeared to deal a major blow to the proponents of sex therapy, it is open to so many criticisms that one must look for evidence from elsewhere. For example, although described as a 'controlled study', allocation of subjects to the three groups was not entirely random; thus, subjects without partners were not allocated to sex therapy. The nature of the sex therapy programme was unclear; treatment sessions were apparently provided every two to three weeks, which most therapists would not regard as a satisfactory schedule. Furthermore, it is unclear what the non-specific treatment was, although it was said that subjects given treatment attended for the same amount of time as those in the other groups. Finally, the measures used to assess outcome were very poor.

A more sophisticated evaluation of sex therapy for couples with a range of sexual problems was conducted by Mathews and colleagues (1976). They compared three forms of treatment: (i) a modified Masters and Johnson approach; (ii) treatment by self-help instructions and very limited therapist contact; and (iii) systematic desensitization plus counselling. Differences in outcome between couples in the three treatment groups were limited, but consistent trends were found at the end of treatment and four months later, favouring the modified Masters and Johnson approach. It is interesting to note in passing that there were a few couples in the group which received self-help instructions and limited therapist contact who did extremely well. One criticism of this study is that the heterogenous nature of the couples and their problems may have obscured more conclusive results.

Everaerd (1977) also compared sex therapy with systematic desensitization in the treatment of two groups of couples: (i) those in which the women experienced orgasmic dysfunction, and (ii) those in which the men had erectile dysfunction. In the first group of couples, the modified Masters and Johnson approach produced much more rapid improvement than systematic desensitization, such that after 12 sessions, five out of 12 couples who received sex therapy had successfully completed treatment whereas none of the other couples had done so. However, at the six-month follow-up, all significant differences between the groups had disappeared. In the second group of couples, in which the men had erectile difficulties, both forms of treatment had only weakly positive effects, there being no difference between the effects of the two approaches either at the end of treatment or at the six month follow-up. Unfortunately, only scanty details of the treatment methods are provided so that critical examination of the study is impossible. Nevertheless, when this study is considered together with that of Ansari (1976) and the follow-up study of Levine and Agle (1978), it raises the important question of how effective sex therapy is for couples with erectile dysfunction. However, in the light of new findings concerning physical causes of erectile problems (Wagner and Green 1981), one suspects that an important factor is inaccurate diagnosis of psychogenic dysfunction in many cases. Certainly, in our clinic, where very careful screening of such cases is carried out, most couples in which the men have erectile dysfunction have a relatively good outcome.

Dow (1983) compared the effectiveness of a modified Masters and Johnson programme with that of treatment by self-help booklets and limited therapist contact (once-weekly telephone conversations) for couples with a range of sexual difficulties. The results of this study are very interesting. First, the couples in which the women had problems of 'sexual unresponsiveness' had a much better outcome with sex therapy than those who received self-help; in fact those in the latter group showed no noticeable improvement. This result may have reflected the high incidence of general relationship difficulties found in couples of this kind, for which marital counselling will often be necessary. Secondly, the couples in which the women had vaginismus had a generally favourable outcome, irrespective of the mode of treatment. Thirdly, those with premature ejaculation as a problem responded poorly to either treatment. This finding is difficult to understand as it is in conflict with general clinical findings concerning the response of premature ejaculation to sex therapy, and also to self-help (Lowe and Mikulas 1975). Finally, sex therapy had a marked beneficial effect on the measures of general marital adjustment, which was not found in the couples in the self-help group.

The general conclusion from these studies is that there is supportive evidence for the superiority of sex therapy compared with other forms of treatment or no treatment at all. In none of the studies, however, was the superiority over other forms of treatment overwhelming. In addition, the effectiveness of sex therapy varies according to the nature of the presenting problem. There is a clear need for further carefully controlled treatment studies.

EVALUATION OF MODIFICATIONS OF THE ORIGINAL MASTERS AND JOHNSON PROGRAMME

Single therapists versus co-therapists

Treatment by male and female co-therapists was an integral

component of the original Masters and Johnson approach. This parameter of sex therapy has been the subject of several investigations. Apart from the study by Mathews *et al.* (1976) noted above, which suggested that sex therapy provided by co-therapists was slightly more effective than when provided by one therapist, all the other investigations have failed to demonstrate any superiority of co-therapy over treatment provided by single therapists (Crowe *et al.* 1981; Clement and Schmidt 1983; Mathews *et al.* 1983; LoPiccolo 1983). An interesting additional finding in the study of Mathews *et al.* (1983) was that men reported more ease of sexual expression when taking part in treatment with only one therapist.

The lack of difference in effectiveness between co-therapy and single-therapist treatment does not mean that co-therapy may not have some advantages. In the treatment of very difficult couples, two therapists may be able to handle complex issues better than one therapist; and in training of therapists, an inexperienced therapist could work alongside an expert. However, in routine clinical practice, treatment by one therapist seems more efficient, especially in terms of economical use of therapists' time.

An additional finding by Crowe and colleagues (1981) concerning single therapists was that there was no interactive effect on outcome between the sex of the therapist and that of the presenting partner. However, in clinical practice there appear to be some couples for whom either a male therapist or a female therapist seems more appropriate. In some cases it appears that one partner would benefit from receiving special support and understanding from a therapist of the same sex (Arentewicz and Schmidt 1983).

Frequency of treatment sessions

In their original approach, Masters and Johnson arranged treatment sessions on a daily basis, seven days per week, with the aim of completing treatment within three weeks. This intensity of treatment is beyond the capacity of most therapists, as it is incompatible with their other clinical and personal demands, and would be unacceptable to most couples. The results of two studies support the use of a less intensive schedule. Clement and Schmidt (1983) found that twice-weekly treatment sessions resulted in better immediate outcome than daily treatment, although this difference had disappeared one year after treatment ended. A study by Heiman and LoPiccolo (1983) indicated that weekly treatment sessions were more effective than daily sessions for couples in which the men had erectile dysfunction or the woman had secondary orgasmic dysfunction. The authors suggested that this may have reflected the longer time course needed for resolution of general relationship difficulties which often accompany these two types of dysfunction. Two other studies have compared weekly with less frequent treatment sessions. Carney *et al.* (1978) found little difference between weekly and monthly sessions in the treatment of couples in which the women had impaired sexual interest. There was, however, some suggestion that the men may have benefited more from the monthly treatment. In another study of couples in which the women had impaired sexual interest, Mathews *et al.* (1983) found that the women appeared to benefit more from weekly rather than monthly treatment sessions, whereas the men were happier with monthly sessions.

Thus there is some evidence in favour of weekly treatment sessions, especially for women. Further research is required concerning the interesting suggestion that there may be a differential sex effect, with men favouring monthly sessions. This has so far only been investigated in couples in which the women had problems concerning their level of sexual interest.

Self-help treatments
There would clearly be considerable savings in therapists' time if sex therapy, or some aspects of it, could be provided in a self-help form. The most obvious means of providing self-help treatment is through instruction manuals, a form of treatment sometimes referred to as 'bibliotherapy'. There have been a few investigations of such an approach with couples which suggest that it may have a place in the management of certain types of uncomplicated problems.

Reference has already been made to two such studies. In the first, by Mathews and colleagues (1976), self-help (instruction manuals) with limited therapist contact (five treatment sessions, including an assessment and a 'round-table' meeting) produced inferior results to sex therapy. However, a few couples in the self-help group did well. Unfortunately, the authors did not indicate which types of sexual problems responded to self-help. In the second study, Dow (1983) found that self-help treatment combined with weekly telephone contact with the therapist was less effective than sex therapy in the treatment of couples with a variety of sexual problems. Surprisingly, however, vaginismus responded equally well to both forms of treatment. General relationship problems were not improved by self-help treatment.

Lowe and Mikulas (1975) studied ten couples in which the men had premature ejaculation. Their treatment consisted of a self-help manual and twice-weekly brief telephone contact. Considerable improvements in ejaculatory control were found after three weeks on the programme. Five of the couples served as controls, being placed on a waiting-list for three weeks before entering the same treatment programme. While no improvement occurred while on the waiting-list, the problems with this form of control group have already been noted (p. 202). However, the changes in ejaculatory control found in this study were marked. It is pertinent to note that the couples were selected for absence of any interpersonal problems which might have required special attention.

Similar findings for couples in which the men had premature ejaculation were obtained by Zeiss (1978). He compared totally self-administered treatment, using a treatment manual, with, secondly, self-administered treatment and brief weekly telephone contacts, and thirdly, therapist-administered treatment. None of the couples in the entirely self-administered treatment group were successful, most giving up the programme early on. However, the couples in the other two groups did much better, with those who had self-administered treatment and limited therapist contact having a similar outcome to those who received the standard treatment. Again it should be noted that none of the couples had gross interpersonal difficulties.

McMullen and Rosen (1979) reported that women with primary total orgasmic dysfunction responded well to a six-week self-help masturbation training programme, although the women had to attend a clinic weekly to obtain instructions for each stage of the programme. The positive gains from treatment transferred to the women's sexual relationships with their partners in about half the successful cases. This was most likely to occur if the partners did not have sexual difficulties themselves.

It appears that self-help treatment can be useful for some couples with premature ejaculation or primary orgasmic dysfunction, provided they do not have interpersonal difficulties. Self-help treatment must be supported by contact with a therapist, even if this consists of brief but regular telephone contact. Considerable care obviously must be paid to the design of the self-help manuals that are used.

CONCLUSIONS

The immediate results of sex therapy obtained in routine clinical practice are not as good as those originally reported by Masters and Johnson. Nevertheless, the results are reasonable, with approximately two-thirds of couples having a satisfactory outcome. Less information is available concerning the longer-term outcome of sex therapy. Benefits from therapy are sustained in many cases, although relapse may be more common in couples presenting with either impaired sexual interest or erectile dysfunction. In a fairly large proportion of couples who respond poorly to sex therapy, the partners will eventually separate. This presumably reflects the fact that their relationship will generally have been less satisfactory at the outset than that of couples who do well.

Investigations of factors which might help predict the outcome of therapy have mostly been limited by being retrospective. However, apart from the nature of the sexual problem, the following factors appear to be related to outcome; the quality of the general relationship, current psychopathology, motivation (with perhaps the man's motivation being especially important), the duration of the sexual problem, a couple's previous sexual adjustment, the extent of sexual attraction between partners, and the progress made early in treatment.

Most controlled studies have demonstrated that sex therapy is superior to other forms of treatment. In general, treatment by a single therapist seems to be as effective as that provided by two therapists. A weekly schedule of treatment sessions is better than more intensive treatment, although there is some suggestion that in couples receiving help for the woman's impaired sexual interest the men may favour less frequent contact with the therapist.

Self-help treatments have a place in the treatment of some couples with straightforward problems, uncomplicated by interpersonal difficulties. Self-help alone, however, is often insufficient; there must also be regular brief contact with the therapist.

14

Further therapeutic approaches

Having considered sex therapy with couples in detail we can now turn our attention to other treatment approaches. Although Masters and Johnson initially provided help for a few dysfunctional men without partners by enlisting the assistance of surrogate partners (Masters and Johnson 1970), they eventually abandoned this highly controversial approach. For some time, considerable pessimism surrounded the question of whether individuals with sexual problems could be helped on their own. Recent innovations, however, mean that effective therapy with individuals is now often possible. Some of the methods of treatment currently available for the individual with sexual difficulties will be described in the first part of this chapter.

Treatment in groups has been another development in this field. Group treatment was introduced partly in the interests of economy, but also to enhance the therapeutic process in the management of certain sexual difficulties. It has mostly been used for individuals with sexual problems, but in some places group treatment of couples is available. Treatment in groups is the topic of the second part of this chapter.

Not all couples or individuals who seek help for sexual disorders require a full sex therapy programme. Many can be helped by brief counselling. This is especially so in primary care. Although family doctors see a fair number of patients for whom sex therapy is necessary, they see many times more people with sexual difficulties who require advice, encouragement, and sexual education, or advice on self-help. Brief counselling is discussed in the third part of this chapter.

In the final section we will consider the type of help that may be provided for people who have sexual difficulties because of physical disorders. Many of the principles of sex therapy can successfully be used to help with the sexual problems of the physically disabled. In addition, there are other procedures that may meet the needs of some disabled people.

TREATMENT OF INDIVIDUALS

Individual treatment is usually indicated because of absence of a partner. However, sometimes one partner is unwilling to be involved in treatment, or cannot attend treatment sessions. An individual approach is then occasionally helpful. Furthermore, there are some sexual problems which may be more easily treated on an individual basis, at least initially. This is often the case for women with primary orgasmic dysfunction and for men with primary ejaculatory failure.

First, the sexual difficulties of women for which an individual approach can be helpful will be considered. Problems concerning levels of sexual interest can rarely be tackled on an individual basis, unless they are the result of either neurotic difficulties, such as anxiety or depressive states, which may respond to individual psychological approaches and/or medication; or physical disorders which will respond to medication (e.g. hypogonadal states).

Orgasmic dysfunction

The treatment of primary orgasmic dysfunction was greatly improved by the introduction of methods in which masturbation has a central role (Nairne and Hemsley 1983). The rationale for this is that many women experience orgasm for the first time through masturbation, and that the proportion of women who are consistently orgasmic with masturbation is far greater than the proportion consistently orgasmic in sexual intercourse (Kinsey *et al.* 1953). In addition to being valuable in helping women without partners, this approach can also be incorporated in the treatment of couples in which the woman is non-orgasmic, either as part of the conjoint programme, or, initially, through individual therapy with the woman alone.

The programme that will be considered is essentially that

introduced by LoPiccolo and Lobitz (1972), and described in detail in a book by Heiman, LoPiccolo, and Lopiccolo (1976). The purpose of this programme is to convey not just the mechanics of masturbation, but to help a woman who has negative feelings about either her body, especially her genitals, or her sexuality, to become more at ease with herself. A powerful factor in the masturbation training programme is the way it helps in the identification of negative or distorted attitudes, which can then be explored further, using some of the techniques described in Chapter 9. It also includes educational components, as discussed in Chapter 10.

When a woman receives individual therapy of this kind it is preferable if the therapist is also a woman, partly because of the potentially erotic nature of the therapeutic interaction. For this reason, male therapists offering this treatment should be extremely cautious.

Before the programme is introduced, the woman must be carefully assessed, covering the areas described in Chapter 6. In particular the therapist should evaluate the woman's attitude to her body, especially her genitals, and to masturbation. Very often the woman must be helped to explore any negative feelings about masturbation before she begins the programme. Provision of some facts about masturbation often helps; for example, that probably as many as 85 per cent of women masturbate at some stage in their lives, and that women who have masturbated seem less often to have sexual difficulties in their relationships. A female therapist can also have an important permission-giving role in suggesting that the woman should allow herself the pleasure of masturbation.

The masturbation training programme is usually introduced gradually, including the following stages:

1. *General self-examination.* This is indicated if the woman has negative feelings about her body. She should choose times when she feels relaxed, and can ensure privacy, and then spend a little while examining herself generally while naked. A useful suggestion is to ask her to identify three aspects of her body which she likes and three which she dislikes. This may help her develop a more rational appraisal of herself. Her attitudes towards her body should then be discussed with the therapist.

2. *Genital self-examination.* Next, the woman is asked to spend

time examining her genital area. She should first do this with a hand-mirror, and try to find the various parts of her genitals which have previously been pointed out by the therapist in a diagram or, preferably, a photograph. She should identify the labia majora and minora, the entrance to her vagina and her clitoris. Resistance may occur at this stage, and is often because the woman thinks that her genitals are unattractive, or that 'one should not touch oneself down there'. Some women become anxious because their genitals do not look exactly the same as those shown in books. The therapist should explain that the appearance of female genitals varies greatly from one woman to another. The woman is asked to repeat this self-examination on at least three occasions, or until she finds she can do it while remaining completely relaxed. She is also encouraged to try to view her genitals as attractive.

Next the woman should explore her genitals with her fingers in order to become familiar with the texture of both the external parts and the inside of her vagina. She is told not to expect to become sexually aroused. Once this stage has been accomplished she should then continue exploring her genitals, but with the aim of locating sensitive areas. In particular she should explore the sensitivity of her clitoris and the surrounding area. When exploring inside her vagina it is helpful if she practises the Kegel exercises at the same time in order to feel the contractions of her vaginal muscles against her fingers.

3. *Kegel exercises.* These exercises were introduced by Kegel (1952) to encourage the development and control of the pubococcygeus muscles which surround the entrance to the vagina. They also help to strengthen all the pelvic floor muscles, and hence are often recommended following childbirth. Apart from improving both the tone of the vaginal muscles, and the woman's control over them, it has also been suggested that these exercises increase orgasmic potential (Graber and Kline-Graber 1980), but this remains unproven (Roughan and Kunst 1981).

If the woman is unsure whether or not she can contract her vaginal muscles, she is asked when next passing urine to try to stop the flow of urine; the pubococcygeus muscles are used to do this. The woman can check that she is contracting the pubococcygeus by placing a finger at the entrance to the vagina where she should be able to feel the muscle contractions.

Once she can contract her vaginal muscles, then, at least three times a day, she should contract them three times as firmly as possible. She might use time cues to remember to do this, such as after going to the toilet, or whenever she has a drink. Next she should extend the number of contractions until eventually she can manage ten at a time.

4. *Masturbation.* Once the woman has located the sensitive parts of her genitals she is asked to concentrate on stimulating these with her fingers. The therapist can discuss different types of masturbation technique. A lotion may be suggested in order to enhance pleasure and prevent soreness. The woman should gradually increase the intensity and duration of masturbation, focusing on any pleasurable sensations that occur.

5. *Adjuncts to masturbation.* The therapist might suggest various means of enhancing sexual arousal during masturbation. If acceptable to the woman, she could be encouraged to read *erotic literature.* She should also be encouraged to use *sexual fantasies.* Some women find it difficult to think of appropriate fantasies, in which case reading a book concerning the sexual fantasies of women (e.g. Friday 1975) may be helpful. This can also provide reassurance about the wide range of fantasies which women find arousing.

If the woman has not experienced orgasm after a few weeks of regular masturbation, the therapist should discuss the question of her purchasing a *vibrator.* The round-headed 'body-massager' type of vibrator is better for this purpose than a phallic-shaped vibrator. The vibrator may be applied either directly to the sensitive parts of the genitals (and to other parts of the body), or indirectly, by placing it over the fingers or over clothing. Some women find that spraying a jet of water from a shower onto their genitals is highly arousing (Barbach 1974). Most women who do not experience orgasm through masturbation alone do so with the help of a vibrator. However, some women express anxieties about using one. A common fear is that if orgasm occurs with a vibrator the woman might become 'hooked' on it. She should be reassured that once she can experience orgasm using a vibrator she will find that she gradually needs to use it less and less. Another anxiety is that a vibrator is an unnecessary sexual aid which will reduce sexuality to a solely mechanical procedure. The woman should be encouraged to view this as a temporary measure to help her overcome her difficulty.

It is not uncommon for a woman to report that she regularly gets highly aroused with masturbation, but reaches a point at which she feels herself 'switch off'. This loss of arousal may result from any one of several fears, which the therapist must help the woman explore. These include anxiety about what will happen during orgasm, and fear of loss of control, or of defaecation or urination. One measure which has been suggested as a means of overcoming such fears is for the woman to *role-play* at home how she thinks she will behave during orgasm (LoPiccolo and Lobitz 1972).

Once the woman can experience orgasm, which is the outcome in most cases (LoPiccolo and Lobitz 1972; Barbach 1974), she should be encouraged to continue masturbating from time to time. Suggestions should also be made concerning how she can transfer to a sexual relationship what she has learned on her own (p. 141). There is good evidence that this type of programme is an effective addition to the programme described in earlier chapters for the treatment of couples in which the woman experiences orgasmic dysfunction. (Munjack *et al.* 1976; Riley and Riley 1978). However, some men are anxious about their partners first learning to experience orgasm with masturbation, because this undermines their own sense of sexual competence. This issue must be explored with both partners before such a programme begins.

Vaginismus

Vaginismus is a problem which primarily affects a woman's relationship with a partner, and is therefore best managed in the context of conjoint therapy. However, occasionally a woman without a partner presents asking for help with this problem, having discovered it during a relationship which has subsequently broken up (possibly as a result of the problem). Although there is no empirical evidence, it seems reasonable to help such a woman in the ways described below and so prepare her for a future relationship. One step is to encourage her to become familiar with her genitals, using the approach suggested above for the treatment of orgasmic dysfunction. A vaginal examination, during which her fears are discussed and she is helped to relax, can be helpful. She should also be taught the Kegel exercises (p. 218). In addition, she should regularly practise inserting one or two fingers into her vagina. An important landmark for such a woman can be the use of tampons, which she is unlikely to have been able to use previously. Graded dilators, whose use was discussed earlier (p. 144), might also be suggested.

Once this programme has been accomplished, the woman should be encouraged to keep practising what she has learned, and also counselled on how to try to have sexual intercourse with a future partner. She should not expect immediate success, but should encourage her partner to take things slowly, preferably explaining to him beforehand the nature of her difficulty.

Premature ejaculation
This problem is also best treated in conjoint therapy, but men without partners often seek help for premature ejaculation. Some of the techniques suggested earlier (p. 148) can be used to help the individual with this problem. A useful approach incorporates a masturbation training programme. The therapist should explain that rapid masturbation may have primed the man to ejaculate rapidly when with a partner (p. 37), and that it would be helpful if the man could learn to reverse this tendency.

First, the man should prolong masturbation until he can last 15 minutes before ejaculating. He should focus on the pleasurable sensations induced by masturbation, and also notice variations in his level of arousal. He should particularly try to identify the point of inevitability after which ejaculation cannot be prevented (p. 20). Often ejaculation has occurred so rapidly before a man enters treatment that he has never been aware of this point. Once he can prolong masturbation quite easily for 15 minutes using a dry hand, the man is then asked to use a lubricant, such as baby lotion. This will probably accelerate his arousal, and be more akin to sensations during sexual intercourse. Again he should aim to prolong masturbation for 15 minutes before ejaculating. Prolongation of masturbation may help him develop the cognitive skills which presumably allow other men to prolong sexual activity. He can make this more realistic by fantasizing sexual activity with a partner while masturbating. An important factor in successful treatment is to develop full awareness of sexual sensations and levels of sexual arousal.

The man can also be instructed in the stop-start or squeeze techniques (p. 148). Reading material, such as a general book on sexuality (e.g. Delvin 1974), and one specifically concerned with sexuality of men (e.g. Zilbergeld 1978), may improve his sexual knowledge and correct sexual myths.

Finally, the man should be advised, if he feels able, to explain his difficulty to a future sexual partner, and to enlist her general co-operation so that he can use the stop-start or squeeze techniques if necessary.

Erectile dysfunction

It is doubtful whether a great deal can be achieved in individual therapy with a man who experiences erectile difficulties when with a partner, because the problem is usually the result of specific anxieties about sexual situations. Probably the most that can be done is to help the man develop more confidence in his sexual ability. He can be taught to practise during masturbation the waxing and waning exercise which was described earlier (p. 148). Fantasizing sexual activity in which he retains his erection should be encouraged. He might also read the books mentioned above for the individual with premature ejaculation, especially Zilbergeld's (1978).

The main strategy in treatment is to explore the anxieties that sexual activity with a partner creates, and to discuss his approach to future sexual relationships. He should avoid rushing into a physical relationship with a new partner, but try to allow it to develop gradually. If he feels confident enough to do so, he might share his problem with his partner and try to enlist her co-operation in helping overcome his anxieties.

Retarded ejaculation

As was noted earlier (p. 152), a man who has never experienced ejaculation, at least while awake, is probably best treated individually in the first instance, even if he has a partner. The aim would be to help him to learn to ejaculate through masturbation. Physical causes for the problem must be ruled out first. If the man experiences nocturnal emissions, a physical cause is unlikely. He should be advised to concentrate on the pleasurable sensations from masturbation, using erotic fantasies and/or sexually stimulating literature or magazines to enhance his arousal. A lotion applied to his penis can also enhance sensations, and reduce the likelihood of soreness. The therapist should explore any difficulties the man has concerning high sexual arousal, such as fear of loss of control. Vibrators do not appear to be as effective in the management of ejaculatory failure as they are in overcoming orgasmic dysfunction in women, but could be tried.

The caution that was expressed earlier concerning the sex of the therapist offering individual treatment to women applies equally in the context of helping men without partners.

TREATMENT IN GROUPS

In recent years, sex therapy has in some centres been conducted in groups. This approach has largely been used for individuals with sexual difficulties, although some therapists have also treated couples in this way. More economical use of therapeutic time has been one reason for this. However, there are other specific advantages of group treatment, as well as some disadvantages, and these are discussed below. We will first examine group treatment of both women and men without partners, and then briefly consider group treatment of couples. The reader who wishes to consult a thorough review of the literature concerning the outcome of group treatment is referred to Mills and Kilmann (1982).

Women

Group treatment has been used most extensively for women with orgasmic dysfunction. In California, Barbach (1974) introduced a group approach for pre-orgasmic women, utilizing the masturbation training programme of LoPiccolo and Lobitz (1972) which was described earlier in this chapter. She introduced the term 'pre-orgasmic' both to avoid the pejorative implications of the term 'non-orgasmic' and to encourage an optimistic attitude towards the outcome of treatment. Her programme, which has been applied successfully by many other therapists in the United States and elsewhere (Mills and Kilman 1982), is outlined below. For a detailed description of how to set up and run pre-orgasmic groups the reader is referred to Barbach (1980).

The aim is to help women begin to experience orgasm, first on their own and subsequently with their partners. For many women this will necessitate a major change in attitude towards masturbation and also towards their right to enjoy sexual pleasure. As with other forms of sex therapy, the programme consists of graduated homework exercises, exploration of attitudes, and sex education.

The programme for pre-orgasmic groups. The treatment schedule used by Barbach consists of ten sessions, with twice-weekly sessions during the first three weeks followed by four weeks of weekly sessions. A follow-up group is usually held approximately three months after the end of treatment. Each group includes between five and ten women. The groups are usually led by two female therapists, although a man might be introduced at some stage to answer specific questions concerning the attitudes of men to the sexuality of women.

During the first session the following homework assignments are suggested. First, each woman is asked to spend time at home examining her body while undressed, preferably in a full-length mirror. As discussed earlier when individual treatment of pre-orgasmic women was considered (p. 217), this exercise is intended to allow a woman to become more comfortable with herself, and to develop a more rational attitude towards her body. Secondly, the women are instructed in the Kegel exercises (p. 218). Thirdly, they are asked to read a book about the health and sexuality of women (Phillips and Rakusen 1978).

During the second session, a few days later, each woman's progress is reviewed. At this stage there is a specific educational input to the programme, to back up what the women have been reading. Female sexual anatomy and sexual response are described (see Chapter 2). The homework assignment this time is for the women to examine their genitals, both with a hand mirror and with their fingers.

In the third session, after discussing their progress, the women are shown a film about masturbation. This often clarifies their attitudes towards masturbation which they are then encouraged to discuss. It also provides an overview of the subsequent stages in the programme. The homework this time is for the women to practise masturbation. However, they are specifically asked *not* to proceed to orgasm. This helps alleviate performance pressures. From the fourth session onwards, each session begins as usual with the women discussing their progress. The homework exercises, which largely concern masturbation, are then individually tailored to the progress of each woman. Now the women are asked to try to reach orgasm. Sexual fantasies, erotic literature, and vibrators are all discussed, and their use encouraged if appropriate (p. 219). During the later sessions in the programme the women are advised how they might transfer what they have learned to a relationship with a partner. Provided her partner will co-operate, a woman might show him how she stimulates herself, and then guide him in both non-genital and genital caressing. Advice is also provided concerning how the woman might stimulate herself during intercourse, and how she can encourage her partner to provide her with manual stimulation.

There appear to be several *advantages* of women receiving help of this kind in groups:

1. The group can provide a *sense of support* between the members. Most women soon realize that their difficulties are similar to those experienced by many other women. It also seems that many women are able to speak with more confidence in a group setting, once they have overcome any initial shyness, than they can in individual therapy. In addition, a woman often derives comfort from knowing that her problems are acceptable to other women.

2. As well as suggestions from the therapists, the women often receive useful *advice and information from other women in the group*.

3. A certain amount of *modelling* may occur in the groups. Thus, some women are likely to follow the lead of others in trying out, for example, different methods of self-stimulation, and when one woman becomes orgasmic this often encourages others to follow her lead.

4. Group treatment is clearly far more *economical* in therapeutic time than individual treatment.

However, there can also be *disadvantages* of this type of treatment. The main one is lack of involvement of a woman's partner in the programme. Some men feel threatened and undermined by this approach, and this may limit generalization of therapeutic gains to the relationship. Many therapists who run pre-orgasmic groups see the partners of the women before the programme begins, and again upon termination, in order to explain the approach and to advise them how they and their partners can gain most from it. Some therapists conduct a few group sessions with the partners which run in parallel with the women's group. Others introduce the partners to the woman's group itself in the later stages of the programme. Further disadvantages of group treatment are that some women find unacceptable the idea of discussing their sexuality with other women, and some fear possible breaches of confidentiality by other group members.

The results of pre-orgasmic groups are generally good. Barbach (1974) reported that 92 per cent of women treated in a series of groups became orgasmic by the end of the ten session programme. Wallace and Barbach (1974) reported follow-up interviews with 17 women eight months after they had participated in the groups. All were orgasmic when their groups ended. At follow-up, only two were not yet orgasmic with their partners, and one woman had not had a partner since receiving treatment. The women also showed several other positive changes, with regard to both their sexuality and their general well-being. This study was limited by lack of a control group.

Leiblum and Ersner-Hershfield (1977) reported less generalization of orgasm to partner stimulation or sexual intercourse in 16 women, 14 of whom had become orgasmic through masturbation by the end of group treatment. However, in a subsequent controlled trial they rather surprisingly found that orgasm with a partner was no more likely among women treated in groups *with* their partners than among women treated in women-only groups (Ersner-Hershfield and Kopel 1979). Ninety-one per cent of all the women were orgasmic through masturbation by the end of treatment and 82 per cent were orgasmic with their partners by the time they were seen for a ten-week follow-up assessment. Pre-orgasmic groups appear to be most successful for women under the age of 35 (Schneidman and McGuire 1976).

Barbach and Flaherty (1980) have described group treatment of women with situational orgasmic dysfunction. Women who either had casual relationships or were in relationships of relatively short duration generally did well. The results were less satisfactory for women in relationships of greater than three years' duration. The authors suggested that additional conjoint therapy might have helped change some well-established patterns in the sexual relationships of the women in long-standing relationships.

Men

Group treatment of men without partners has received less attention than that of women and the results of such treatment are generally inferior, especially for men with erectile dysfunction. Zilbergeld (1975) introduced group treatment for men with either erectile or ejaculatory difficulties. Each group was conducted by a male and a female therapist. They met on 12 occasions, at first weekly, and later on a more widely spaced schedule. As in the women's groups described earlier, therapy included homework assignments, sex education, and regular discussion of each individual's progress. The main homework assignment was masturbation training, as described earlier (p. 221). In addition, the men received relaxation training, and common male sexual myths (Zilbergeld 1978) were discussed. Although specific evaluation of outcome was not reported, Zilbergeld claimed that two-thirds of the men said they had completely achieved their goals by the end of treatment. He also advised other therapists who wished to conduct group treatment to place men with the same type of dysfunction in each group, rather than mixing those with erectile difficulties and those with ejaculatory problems.

A similar approach was used by Lobitz and Baker (1979) in the treatment of men with erectile dysfunction and, although their study was again uncontrolled, they also reported reasonable gains from treatment. However, men with primary situational erectile dysfunction did badly and in these cases the authors recommended a conjoint approach.

The importance of having a control group in evaluative studies was illustrated by Price *et al.* (1981), who allocated men with secondary erectile dysfunction to one of two treatment groups or to a waiting-list control condition. Although the men who underwent group treatment reported improved attitudes to their sexuality and to their problems, no difference was found between their reports of erectile difficulties following treatment and those of the men in the control group at the end of the period on the waiting-list. Price and colleagues attributed the relative lack of success of their treatment groups to either the older age of the men (mean of 45 years) compared with those treated by other workers, or to the lack of attention paid to 'dating-skills' in the groups. The latter suggestion received support from a more successful study by the same team (Reynolds *et al.* 1981) in which social skills training and homework assignments concerning social interaction were incorporated into group treatment of men with secondary erectile dysfunction. The erectile function of these men improved more than that of similar men in a waiting list control group.

Zeiss (1978) reported satisfactory results with a six-session group approach to the treatment of men with premature ejaculation. Their partners did not participate in the groups but were expected to co-operate with sexual and communication exercises between treatment sessions.

Group treatment of men merits further attention and development because sexual dysfunction clinics receive many requests for help from men with sexual difficulties who either do not have partners, or whose partners are unwilling to attend treatment sessions.

Couples

Group treatment of couples with sexual dysfunction has been introduced in two formats. First, sex therapy along the lines already described for treatment of couples has been provided in groups. Secondly, brief intensive programmes spanning one weekend or a similar time period have been used. The latter usually include a largely educational input and examination of attitudes of group members. Little is known about the effectiveness of this second approach, although preliminary studies suggest it may convey some fairly immediate benefits (Leiblum and Rosen 1979; Chesney *et al.* 1981) and that these may increase during the period following the group experience (Blakeney *et al.* 1976).

Provision of sex therapy to couples in groups has received more attention. Some therapists have restricted such treatment to couples with the same presenting problem. For example, Kaplan *et al.* (1974) reported the treatment of four couples in which the men had premature ejaculation. Homework assignments included sensate focus and the stop-start technique (p. 149).

There were six sessions of treatment, each lasting 45 minutes. Two men gained good ejaculatory control by the end of treatment, and the other two had done so two months later. The approach necessitated an average of 1.5 hours of therapist's time per couple, which was far less than the average of seven hours per couple normally needed in the individual treatment of couples. Other therapists have reported reasonable results from group treatment of couples with mixed dysfunctions (e.g. Leiblum *et al.* 1976), although no controlled studies have so far been carried out. McGovern *et al.* (1976) and Golden *et al.* (1978) ran groups in which both partners had sexual difficulties, the men premature ejaculation and the women orgasmic dysfunction. Sex education and advice on improving communication skills and sexual techniques formed the core of treatment. Considerable improvement in the ejaculatory control of the men and the women's orgasmic capacity resulted from treatment in both studies.

There are three important questions concerning how group treatment of couples compares with individual treatment of couples, namely, do the approaches differ in terms of, first, efficacy, secondly, economy, and, thirdly, acceptability? In the study by Golden *et al.* (1978) noted above, group treatment was compared with individual couple treatment, both involving 12 sessions of treatment conducted by co-therapists. Couples in the two conditions had a similar outcome although there was a suggestion of more rapid early progress by those in the groups.

Duddle and Ingram (1980) compared group and individual couple treatment for couples in which the women had the major sexual problems (although women with vaginismus were excluded). The groups, which each included a maximum of five couples, were conducted by co-therapists and met between 10 and 13 occasions. The individual treatment of couples was also provided by co-therapists. Roughly two-thirds in both treatment formats benefitted from treatment.

A tentative answer to the first question posed above appears to be, therefore, that group treatment of couples may be as effective as conjoint treatment. Secondly, group treatment may also be more economical. We noted earlier the time saved through group treatment of couples in which the men had premature ejaculation (Kaplan *et al.* 1974). Duddle and Ingram (1980) reported a significant, but less substantial saving in therapists' time from approximately 4.5 hours/couple in the conjoint format to 3.8 hours/ couple in the group format. However, while group treatment is probably best conducted by co-therapists, the findings of several studies in which treatment of individual couples was just as effectively carried out by one therapist as two have already been discussed (p. 209). The apparent saving in therapeutic time reported by Duddle and Ingram, who had two therapists in both treatment conditions, is therefore probably misleading.

Thirdly, group treatment is certainly less acceptable for most couples. Duddle and Ingram (1980) reported that many couples refused group treatment, presumably because they did not wish to discuss their sexual relationships with other people. A further drawback of group treatment is the problem of confidentiality (which applies to all forms of group treatment). There might also be a danger of attraction between the partners of different couples because of the potentially erotic nature of the therapeutic situation. Finally, therapists conducting groups may find it difficult to allow for the different rates of progress made by each couple.

In conclusion, it appears that group treatment of couples, provided it is carefully organized, offers a useful additional therapeutic approach to sexual problems, but it is unlikely to be suitable for more than a relatively small minority of couples.

BRIEF COUNSELLING

Many couples and individuals who seek help for sexual difficulties do not require sex therapy. This applies to the majority of such people seen in primary care and other medical settings, and some of those who present to sexual dysfunction clinics. Instead, brief counselling is often sufficient (Annon 1974). This does not demand expertise in sex therapy, although this may help. Brief counselling for sexual problems is relevant for doctors and other professional workers in a wide variety of settings. Examples of such settings include primary care, obstetrics and gynaecology, family planning clinics, a variety of general medical and surgical settings (e.g. diabetic and hypertension clinics, breast cancer clinics), psychiatry out-patient clinics, and marriage guidance council offices.

The main strategies employed in brief counselling are:

(1) assessment;	(5) provision of information;
(2) listening;	(6) encouraging communication;
(3) reassurance;	(7) specific suggestions;
(4) permission;	(8) self-help.

Each of these strategies, together with specific examples, is considered below.

Assessment

Before instituting any kind of help the therapist must first carry out an adequate assessment to ensure a reasonable understanding of the problem. However, in brief counselling the assessment usually need not be as extensive as that recommended in sex therapy (Chapter 6). It is often sufficient to have a clear idea of the presenting problem and to know a little about the person's sexual development and current relationship.

Listening

During brief counselling, the therapist should demonstrate a willingness to listen to what the patient wishes to say. The patient's account can be encouraged by, for example, looking attentive and interested, nodding, and, when the patient hesitates, by statements such as 'Tell me more about this', or by repeating some of what the patient last said, e.g. 'You were saying that when you kiss your girlfriend you feel aroused, but at the same time apprehensive'. Careful attention should also be paid to both verbal and non-verbal cues, such as those suggesting anxiety, or signs that the problem may be more extensive or different from the one that was initially presented. Examples of verbal cues are hesitations and slips of the tongue. Examples of non-verbal cues are signs of embarrassment, avoidance of eye contact, and wringing of hands. Occasionally such signs indicate that a person has something particularly important to discuss, such as an affair, anxiety about sexual anatomy, or the acceptability of a particular form of sexual behaviour.

Reassurance

Reassurance is one of the most important strategies in brief counselling. It requires the therapist to have an adequate knowledge of sexuality and common sexual anxieties. The following are four examples of situations in which reassurance may be helpful.

Many men have anxieties about their penis size. A useful means of reassurance is to point out the foreshortening effect when a man looks down at his penis (p. 179). The relative unimportance of penis size for adequate stimulation of a woman during sexual intercourse can also be explained (p. 179).

People sometimes express the fear that they are abnormally highly responsive. For example, a woman might ask if she is abnormal because she is able to respond very rapidly to her partner's sexual advances but has read that women usually respond relatively slowly compared with men. She could be reassured that some women respond faster than others, and that many women are able to respond as quickly as their partners. The therapist might add that the woman and her partner are fortunate in that she is able to respond quickly.

Some couples are worried when the woman's interest in sex has not returned soon after childbirth. Because of the association between childbirth and the onset of sexual problems (p. 64), reassurance is most important at this time. Reassurance that sexual interest usually returns gradually after childbirth, and that there may be a considerable delay before things are back to normal, is likely to be most effective if both partners hear it.

People suffering from depression often worry about their lack of interest in sex. They may be reassured that this is a common feature of depression, as is a general loss of affectional feelings. However, this interest will gradually return as the affective disorder responds to treatment, although interest in sex often returns fairly late during recovery from depression.

Permission

An important first step in brief counselling is to make it clear that sexuality is a legitimate topic for discussion. Many people believe that doctors in particular are not interested in hearing about their patient's sexual difficulties.

More specific examples of situations in which a therapist might be giving permission include encouraging couples to experiment with different sexual positions in order to find one in which the woman receives more effective stimulation; suggesting that a man provides his partner with manual stimulation during sexual intercourse when previously the couple have regarded such stimulation as unnatural; and helping a couple to enjoy freely behaviour which is already part of their sexual repertoire but about which one or both of them feels guilty or anxious. In using such a strategy the therapist must always remember the danger of imposing sexual values on people (p. 244).

Provision of information

Provision of information about sexuality can help improve sexual knowledge and dispel sexual myths. Examples include explaining the importance of the clitoris in sexual stimulation; pointing out to a man that a woman is unlikely to enjoy sexual intercourse if she is unaroused beforehand; dispelling fears that masturbation is harmful; and explaining that there is no physical danger associated with sexual intercourse during menstruation.

A further means of helping improve sexual knowledge is by recommending appropriate reading material. Examples of some suitable books are provided in an Appendix at the end of this book.

Encouraging communication

Earlier it was noted that faulty or absent communication between partners can both cause and maintain sexual difficulties (p. 70). In brief counselling with couples, therapists can often encourage better communication by helping the partners to express their needs and anxieties to each other during counselling sessions. A useful technique is to deflect statements directed to the therapist by one partner towards the other partner. For example, if a man says he thinks that his partner does not like something, the therapist can question whether he has asked her, and, if not, suggest that he does so there and then. The therapist can encourage the couple to persist with such communication by pointing out how this will help avoid misunderstandings and make it easier in future for them to help each other.

Specific suggestions

Components of the sex therapy programme described earlier might be included in brief counselling. For example, a couple in which the man has premature ejaculation, but whose sexual relationship is otherwise satisfactory, might simply be taught the squeeze or stop-start techniques. Similarly, advice can be given on suitable positions for sexual intercourse if a woman experiences dyspareunia on deep penetration as a result of an irremediable physical condition, such as pelvic adhesions (p. 145). Occasionally a couple report that the woman's vagina seems too slack. This might be the result of multiple childbirths. A sensible suggestion is for the woman to practise the Kegel exercises (p. 218). A further suggestion might be for the woman to keep her legs close together once her partner has entered her in order to encompass his penis more tightly.

Specific suggestions must never be made injudiciously, but only when full appraisal of a problem indicates that they are appropriate. For example, to suggest to a 55-year-old woman that she should purchase a vibrator to assist her failing ability to experience orgasm is likely to produce horror, unless the therapist has established that the woman wishes to experiment in order to improve her lovemaking.

Self-help

The limitations of self-help treatments for sexual problems when compared with sex therapy have already been discussed (p. 211). However, it was noted that self-help treatment, when combined with occasional contact with a therapist, even by telephone, can prove effective. Recommending appropriate self-help manuals and books is therefore an important component of brief counselling with some people. This applies especially to women with orgasmic dysfunction (McMullen and Rosen 1979), who may find the book by Barbach (1976) or that written by Heiman *et al.* (1976) helpful. There are several self-help books for couples with a range of sexual difficulties (e.g. Brown and Faulder 1977; Greenwood 1984). Although the efficacy of these has not been tested, they might be worth recommending to couples with sexual problems provided they do not also have major problems in their general relationship.

Clinical experience suggests that brief counselling is often satisfactory in the management of people with relatively uncomplicated sexual problems. The situation should be reviewed a few weeks or months after the counselling in order to ensure that progress has been sustained. This also provides an opportunity for further counselling, or for referral for specialist help if necessary. Brief counselling is sometimes useful before beginning more intensive sex therapy. It may then become apparent that the brief approach is all that is required. In other cases it can clarify the precise nature of the sexual difficulty, and might occasionally provide a useful test of motivation when this is in doubt.

MANAGEMENT OF SEXUAL PROBLEMS ASSOCIATED WITH PHYSICAL DISABILITY

The term 'physical disability' is used here in a very general sense to include, for example, paraplegia resulting from spinal cord injury, hemiplegia associated with stroke or other cerebral damage, and chronic physical disorders, such as diabetes, multiple sclerosis, and arteriosclerosis, which frequently interfere with sexual performance. A review of the effects of these and other physical conditions was provided in Chapter 5. We will not consider all the details of management of sexual difficulties of this kind because this is available elsewhere (e.g. Heslinga 1974). Instead, three broad approaches will be discussed, namely brief counselling, sex therapy, and the use of physical aids.

Brief counselling

For most people who require help for sexual problems resulting from physical disability, brief counselling is probably sufficient. In the previous section we examined the components of this approach. Their application to the specific problems of people with physical disorders will now be discussed.

Listening. Sensitive listening is especially important in dealing with people who suffer from physical disability, because they are often aware of the common adverse attitudes to their sexual difficulties. Some of those who care for disabled people continue to maintain the illusion that disabled persons lack sexuality. Not only is this patently untrue, but it is known that as many as two-thirds of severely disable people encounter problems in fulfilling their sexual needs (Stewart 1978).

Provision of information.   A very important stage in counselling people with sexual problems associated with physical disorders is to explain how their physical condition interferes with sexual response. A significant change in attitude often accompanies the realization that the sexual difficulty is not the result of some decline in masculinity or femininity, but has a recognized and understandable physical basis. Thus the diabetic man who has developed erectile difficulties can blame his illness rather than himself for the problem, and his partner may also be reassured by the knowledge that the difficulty does not mean that he no longer finds her attractive. When providing such information the therapist must also explain how emotional responses of both partners to the problem may have made it worse. For example, the woman's fear that her diabetic partner no longer desired her may have caused her to avoid sexual activity, thereby adding to her partner's anxieties, and these are likely to have exacerbated his erectile difficulties.

Permission.   People with physical disorders often have to make considerable changes in their sexual relationship in order to compensate for the disability. A therapist can often help by encouraging them to experiment with sexual behaviours they might previously have considered taboo. This is very important when a couple are unable to have sexual intercourse because of the disability (e.g. complete erectile dysfunction because of spinal cord transection or sacral nerve damage following a pelvic operation). A therapist might help such a couple to accept that a satisfying and enjoyable sexual relationship need not involve sexual intercourse. Therapists also play a permission-giving role when encouraging, for example, new sexual positions to accommodate to a disability (e.g. the female superior position when a man has had a leg amputated). The danger of imposing unacceptable sexual values on people is as relevant here as when dealing with the able-bodied (p. 244).

Specific suggestions.   There are a wide range of suggestions people with various types of physical disability can use to improve their sexual relationships (see, for example, Heslinga (1974)). A useful general piece of advice, derived from sex therapy, is that couples concentrate particularly on general carressing, as in the sensate focus exercises. This may be particularly helpful for people recovering from serious illness, such as a heart attack, or from major surgery, when there may be anxieties about immediately resuming a full sexual relationship. More specific suggestions include, for example, advice on positions for sexual intercourse for men who experience persistent physical weakness following a stroke (such as the female superior or side-by-side position); techniques of using clothing best to hide the presence of a stoma bag; the advisability of the person who is paraplegic ensuring that his/her bladder and bowels are empty before sexual activity begins; and suggesting to a person with a debilitating disorder that sexual activity might be most successful if it occurs in the morning when he/she is likely to be most alert.

Encouraging communication. Just as is the case with the able-bodied, good sexual adjustment in a couple in which one partner is physically disabled will depend on the ability of the partners to discuss their anxieties and their needs with each other. A therapist might help a disabled person to explain to the partner what type of caressing or stimulation is pleasurable, and what is uncomfortable or even painful. A paraplegic woman, for example, may find that she enjoys being caressed in parts of her body different from those she enjoyed before she suffered her spinal injury. The woman may get little pleasure from her sexual relationship if her partner is unaware of this.

Reassurance. One important way in which a therapist can assist a couple to adjust to physical disability is by helping them accept that sexual satisfaction is not necessarily equated with sexual performance. A great deal of satisfaction can be gained from the sense of intimacy that may accompany a close, trusting physical relationship, even if full sexual response is not feasible for one or even both partners. The therapist should avoid simply telling couples this, but instead, encourage the partners to reassure each other.

Sex therapy
A more extensive approach, incorporating the principles and techniques of sex therapy which were described earlier in this

book, can be very useful in helping couples if emotional factors have played a large part in their poor sexual adjustment to physical disability, or if such factors have resulted in partially impaired performance developing into complete failure or avoidance of sexual activity. This is common in men with conditions such as diabetes and multiple sclerosis, when early difficulties in obtaining or sustaining an erection because of damage to the neural pathways involved in sexual response may cause such anxiety that the erectile problem increases. This type of problem can sometimes be resolved by brief counselling. However, if the psychological factors seem to be well established, a full sex therapy programme is more likely to be effective.

The therapist must initially try to establish the extent to which physical and psychological factors are contributing to the sexual problem. This may not be easy, and both the therapist and the couple may have to accept considerable initial uncertainty. This should be discussed during the formulation (Chapter 7). The situation will usually become clearer as sex therapy proceeds.

The approach with couples with physical disability is usually very similar to that employed in sex therapy with the able-bodied. The aims of therapy include:

(1) helping the partners to adjust their attitudes so that they can accept that sexual intimacy need not depend on sexual performance, and assisting them to adopt a less genitally orientated approach to sexual expression;

(2) encouraging them to maximize their erotic pleasure; for example, if erectile dysfunction is thought to be partial the woman should be encouraged to provide more genital stimulation for her partner, as this may result in considerable improvement in his erection, especially if he can focus his attention on his genital sensations;

(3) identification of attitudes which may be interfering with sexual interaction or preventing the uninhibited enjoyment of erotic pleasure (using the techniques described in Chapter 9);

(4) improving the partners' sexual knowledge if there are important areas of ignorance, as well as supplying specific information concerning the effects of the physical disorder;

(5) assisting the couple to adjust to any limitation imposed by the physical disorder;

(6) if indicated, preparing the couple to accept the eventual

situation which may develop in the case of a progressive physical disorder, such as diabetes or multiple sclerosis. This usually means helping them enjoy non-coital sexual activity as fully as possible.

This type of approach to sexual problems related to physical disorders has so far not been subjected to controlled evaluation. However, the experience of the author, and of other writers (Renshaw 1978; Schiavi 1980), suggests that it can be very successful. It is an important new application of sex therapy which now requires both further development and evaluation.

Sexual aids

These have a relatively small but nevertheless useful role in the management of some sexual problems associated with physical disorders. Only two types of sexual aids will be considered here, namely penile prostheses and the penile ring, both of which are sometimes used for erectile dysfunction. A review of other types of sexual aids has been provided by Rhodes (1975).

Penile prostheses. There is now an extensive literature on the use of implanted penile prostheses (reviewed by Wagner (1981c)). There are two main types of implant. The first is a fairly simple device consisting of two flexible silastic rods which are implanted in the penis, one into each corpus cavernosum. This produces a flexible erection which is sufficiently rigid for sexual intercourse. Although the erection is permanent, it can be hidden under clothing quite easily, especially if placed against the lower abdomen. The second type consists of a pair of inflatable penile implants which are connected to a reservoir lying in the scrotum and a small pump placed under the skin of the lower abdomen. The system contains a radiopaque fluid, and the inflatable tubes are inflated through pressure applied to the pump. Thus the erection is not permanent. However, the surgical procedure necessary to implant this type of prosthesis is more complicated, and there is a significant risk of post-operative infection.

At present the indications for penile implants are not altogether clear, although they are being used fairly extensively in the USA. They may have a place in the management of men with permanent erectile dysfunction, resulting, for example, from diabetes or priapism. However, they should probably only be considered if the man has had reasonable previous sexual adjustment, and if he and his partner have made efforts to develop their sexual relationship since the development of the erectile disorder. Very careful assessment should therefore precede any suggestion that such a device might be useful. A couple will usually need counselling both in preparation for, and subsequent to the operation.

Although penile implants may occasionally be useful, they have several potential disadvantages, in addition to the risk of infection. First, they are expensive. Secondly, they do not enhance a man's sensations of arousal or orgasm. Thirdly, some women respond poorly to them, occasionally because they fear causing damage if they stimulate the penis. In addition, some women have reported that they dislike being uncertain whether or not they are arousing their partners.

At present, therefore, the role of penile implants in the management of erectile dysfunction caused by physical disorders is uncertain. It is probably best to explore the possibility of helping a couple adjust to a non-coital sexual relationship before considering the use of an implant.

Penile ring.   This is a roughly rectangular ebonite hinged device which is fitted so that it encircles the base of the penis and scrotum. One form of the device incorporates electro-galvanic plates which, the manufacturers have claimed, generate a small electric current which stimulates penile blood flow and encourages erection. They also recommend that this device is worn throughout much of the day to facilitate erectile response when sexual activity occurs. However, no difference in effectiveness was found between this form and a more simple version, which lacked the electro-galvanic plates, when tested in a double-blind cross-over trial with 40 men suffering from erectile dysfunction (Cooper 1974). Both versions of the ring produced significant improvements in erectile function. The ring probably acts by having a mild tourniquet effect, reducing blood flow from the penis and also compressing the bulbar part of the corpus spongiosum. It need only be used, therefore, during sexual activity. For couples who are not bothered by the somewhat unattractive appearance of this device, it can be of considerable assistance. It is probably most useful for men who can still obtain partial erections. Cheap penile constriction rings as sold in sex shops are not recommended because they can be dangerous.

CONCLUSIONS

Several developments which have broadened the scope of sex therapy, and some other therapeutic approaches to sexual difficulties, have been considered in this chapter. One of the most significant developments has been the introduction of effective methods of helping individuals with sexual problems. This has been a very welcome advance because, previously, individuals who sought help without partners were usually told that they could not be helped until they had found a cooperative partner. Some important questions still remain, however, most of which concern the extent to which gains from individual therapy generalize to subsequent relationships, especially when men receive such help.

Treatment in groups represents another important development. It has been used extensively for women with orgasmic dysfunction for whom it is extremely effective. Less is known at present about the effectiveness of group treatment for men with sexual difficulties. Group treatment, both for men and for women, can help save much valuable therapeutic time, and may have other advantages, including support and advice between group members. The role of group treatment for couples is less clear. Many couples refuse to enter group treatment when offered it, preferring the greater privacy of conjoint treatment.

Brief counselling can be an effective approach to many sexual difficulties, especially those encountered in primary care and specialist medical settings. The ability to provide such counselling does not demand expertise in sex therapy. The strategies which are used in brief counselling are straightforward, provided that the therapist has a reasonable understanding of human sexuality.

The sexual problems that often accompany physical disability or chronic illness have been grossly neglected in the past. Fortunately, they are now beginning to receive some attention. Brief counselling, including specific advice relevant to the special needs of those with physical disability, is often sufficient, especially if emotional factors are not prominent. When sexual dysfunction is the result of both physical and emotional factors, sex therapy may be more effective. Sexual aids have a small but nevertheless significant role in the management of some sexual problems, especially permanent erectile dysfunction.

15

Concluding comments

Chapter 1 began with some reflections on how the introduction of sex therapy at the beginning of the 1970s marked a major change in the way that people construed sexual problems. They ceased to be regarded as superficial symptoms of deep-seated neurotic problems, but were instead described in terms of impaired learning of sexual skills. This meant that help which consisted of training new skills, education and counselling, was usually beneficial and could be provided through relatively brief therapy. Once this optimistic view led to the increasing availability of therapeutic facilities, vast numbers of people began to seek help for their sexual difficulties. Sex therapy was, at first, largely only available for couples with sexual problems, but, as therapists became more innovative, many individuals with sexual problems were also able to receive help. In previous chapters, the treatment of both couples and individuals with sexual problems has been described in detail. In this final chapter, we will consider some aspects of this field which previously only received brief mention, including the more important clinical and research needs.

The role of cultural factors in the presentation of sexual problems and in sex therapy

Attitudes and values concerning human sexuality have undergone vast changes in recent years, and these have had a major influence on how many people regard their personal sexuality and their sexual relationships. While some of these changes have resulted in greater freedom to enjoy sex for many individuals, they have also presented some people with new pressures which have had implications for their perception of sexual problems and the need to seek help for them.

The most dramatic changes have concerned female sexuality, with the women's liberation movement encouraging women to take more responsibility for their sexuality and also to expect more pleasure from their sexual relationships. This has undoubtedly provided major benefits for many women. For others, this change has caused them to find fault with their sexuality, which has been reflected in the large number of women seeking help for sexual problems, particularly concerning their enjoyment of sex. At the same time, some women have perhaps become unnecessarily dissatisfied, especially as a result of the portrayal of sex by the media. The constant reminders that women should be sexual and attractive, with slimness an important part of this, has caused some women to experience sexual problems which otherwise might not have existed. Many women are now dissatisfied with their body image, and increasingly therapists are emphasizing in sex therapy the need for people, especially women, to develop more accepting attitudes towards their bodies generally, as it has become obvious that poor self-image is a major factor contributing to sexual dysfunction.

At the same time, attitudes towards male sexuality have also undergone significant, if less dramatic, changes. The man's role in being caring, showing affection and tenderness, is still played down, yet many of the complaints of women concern the failure of their partners to demonstrate these qualities. One important component in sex therapy, therefore, is the emphasis on giving and receiving of pleasure through the sensate focus exercises. Another is on communication, with men as well as women being encouraged to tell their partners about their feelings and needs.

Ethical aspects of sex therapy

While carefully conducted sex therapy undoubtedly helps counter some of the pressures that have arisen out of current attitudes towards sexuality, it is possible for therapists to increase such pressures. The value system implied by sex therapy, at least on the face of it, is that the goal of all sexual relationships should be a freedom to enjoy whatever is pleasurable, totally open communication about all sexual matters, and a liberal attitude towards sexuality. This is fallacious—the most important criterion must be what each individual wants, not what he or she is pressurized into thinking is necessary in order to conform with a stereotyped model of satisfactory sexuality, nor, especially, what a therapist deems as being the most satisfactory type of sexual relationship.

It is essential to establish with every couple or individual in therapy the best programme likely to help them achieve their desired objectives. Quite often, one or both partners will object to trying something which the therapist has suggested. The therapist should not put pressure on them to follow a particular suggestion, but should establish the strength of the objection, perhaps explore its basis, and then, if the suggestion is clearly unacceptable, try to find some other approach to the problem. When resistance to a suggestion appears to relate to the development of the sexual problem, the therapist should help the couple to understand this, but not try to persuade them that they must do what has been suggested. There will sometimes be disagreement between partners about the desirability of a particular form of sexual behaviour. Again, the therapist should not try to decide what is best, but should aim to help the partners explore their different views to see if some agreement can be reached, which may often be a compromise.

Problems not helped by sex therapy

Sex therapy is not a panacea; there are many people with sexual problems for whom it is unhelpful. It is not possible, at present, to draw a clear distinction between those who will benefit and those who will not. In several places in this book, emphasis has been placed on the important influence that serious interpersonal difficulties between partners can have on outcome. People with severe problems concerning intimacy are also often difficult to help. Their problems are an exception to what was said at the beginning of this chapter, having often been lifelong and probably having their origins in highly disturbed relationships within the family during childhood. As Kaplan (1979) has noted, intensive psychotherapy aimed at exploring the nature of these early relationships may be the treatment of choice in the first instance, following which effective sex therapy might be possible. This approach requires further investigation and remains conjectural at present.

Sex therapy and the disabled

Although some people's problems will not be helped by sex therapy, there are many other people who might benefit but for whom such help is rarely available. The physically disabled are the most important group. Clinical experience has shown that therapy with people with physical disability is often very fruitful, and in many instances can be briefer than therapy with people whose problems are entirely emotional or interpersonal in origin. This is an important area of clinical need. Very often there is a great reluctance to explore the sexuality of people with physical disabilities; hence the myth of the sexless invalid persists. Couples in which the men have developed diabetic erectile dysfunction provide an excellent example. Those in which one or other partner has undergone mutilating surgery are another. The development of therapeutic approaches to sexual problems resulting from physical disability, along the lines suggested in the previous chapter, offers a major clinical challenge.

The mentally handicapped are another large group of people whose sexual difficulties have hardly been explored. Their problems raise a host of other issues, including those concerning self-control, consent, and the extent to which staff in institutions should limit the sexual freedom of patients.

Meeting the demand for sex therapy

Once sex therapy became available, the extent of the demand for help with sexual problems soon became apparent. Anyone who has set up a sexual problems clinic in the UK will confirm that the pressure of referrals soon outgrows the amount of therapy time available. In some clinics, long waiting-lists are allowed to develop; in others the therapists avoid long waiting-lists by being highly selective. The situation in the USA appears to be rather different in that many more therapists are available, especially for people who can pay for their therapy. The demand in the UK is clearly far greater than can be met with the facilities available at present. This is partly because the development of sex therapy clinics has usually depended upon the enthusiasm of individuals rather than being part of health service policy. This is regrettable, particularly in the light of the distress that sexual problems may cause parents and other adults, and because of the very damaging effects that parental disharmony can have on children.

Part of the problem is that the place of sex therapy in medicine is unclear. Some people think it has no place at all. Others think it should be part of gynaecology or family planning; others think it should be in the realm of psychiatry and clinical psychology. It is hardly surprising, therefore, that sex therapy gains the serious attention of none of these fields. Fortunately, the National Marriage Guidance Council in the UK has put a vast effort into training marriage guidance counsellors to help with their clients' sexual problems as well as their general relationship difficulties (Heisler 1983). However, Marriage Guidance will never be able to meet the needs of all the people with sexual problems who are likely to seek help. Moreover, medical knowledge is necessary for the treatment of the sexual problems of some groups of people.

With the increasing number of physical causes of sexual problems now being discovered, one important question concerns how people working in non-medical settings can ensure that they are not overlooking physical pathology. The safest approach would be to have ready access to an interested physician and a gynaecologist. A general practitioner might be another source of medical advice. Regular meetings with a medical colleague at which cases with the greatest risk of physical pathology (especially men with erectile disorders and women with dyspareunia) could be discussed would be one safeguard.

Training in sex therapy

An important question is how people can obtain training in sex therapy. One approach developed in the UK by the National Marriage Guidance Council has been to train many counsellors by having an inexperienced therapist work as a cotherapist with a more experienced counsellor, and also by often having a further trainee act as an observer in treatment sessions. The author has trained therapists using a different approach (Hawton 1980). Between seven and ten trainee therapists meet weekly in a supervision group. After a few induction sessions, each trainee individually takes on for treatment a couple who have already been assessed for suitability by the group leader. Each trainee is then carefully supervised throughout treatment, all the couples being discussed each week in the supervision group. Trainees are expected to treat at least three consecutive couples before leaving the group. Although this is a smaller number than might be considered ideal, it at least means that the trainees will be able to manage some of the sexual problems they encounter subsequently in the course of their everyday work. The trainees come from a wide variety of disciplines including psychiatry, clinical psychology, general practice, social work, nursing and gynaecology. One prerequisite is that the trainees should have gained some prior experience in counselling. The results obtained by the trainees are satisfactory (Hawton 1980). Trainees who appear to make the most effective therapists are those who are able to adhere to the therapy programme, yet are flexible, and are generally psychologically minded. Both the apprenticeship approach and group supervision of individual trainees appear to be effective methods of training.

Prevention of sexual problems

This book has been about secondary prevention; that is, how to help people who have already developed sexual problems. What about preventing sexual problems in the first place (i.e. primary prevention)? This leads immediately to the controversial topic of sex education. There is little doubt that inadequate sexual knowledge is an important factor in the aetiology of many sexual problems. Some of the people seen today in sexual dysfunction clinics have had no sex education at all, either formal or informal. The educational component of therapy quite often seems to outweigh in importance the other components. Yet there is still a very powerful lobby, both in this country and in the USA, which opposes sex education in schools, usually on the grounds that sex education should be the prerogative of parents. Unquestionably, parents are the major influence on the sexual attitudes of young people and their influence begins very early in life, probably when children first begin genital exploration and fondling (Calderone 1978). Many parents, unfortunately, will have experienced inadequate or nil sex education. How, therefore, are such parents to help their children develop a healthy and informed approach to their own sexuality?

It is the author's opinion that sex education must be taught in schools. The aim should be the achievement of healthy and positive attitudes towards sexuality. Such education should not simply include the topics of physical changes at puberty, menstruation, reproduction, contraception and venereal disease, but also sufficient information about sexual anatomy, response, and behaviour to provide a sound basic understanding of what is known about human sexuality. Furthermore, it should include discussion of how individuals can improve their communication about sex, the importance of each person taking responsibility for his or her own sexuality, and examination of moral and religious aspects of sexuality. Some opponents of sex education in schools feel that it will encourage promiscuity. Commonsense suggests that the opposite would be more likely, and certainly there is no supportive evidence for this fear (Calderone 1978). A good index of whether sex education was successful would, of course, be a decline in the numbers of people seeking help for sexual problems.

The important role of the media in shaping attitudes towards sexuality has already been noted. The media also have a major place in sex education, both of young people and of adults. The numbers of programmes on television about sexuality, and of articles in popular magazines about both male and female sexuality, continue to increase. Those responsible for such programmes and articles should be aware of the extent to which they might help promote healthy and informed attitudes towards sexuality, and the danger of presenting material that might mislead people or impose pressures to live up to arbitrary standards.

Research needs

Research in the field of human sexuality has been of an extremely variable quality. The first need, therefore, is to ensure that the standards of research in this field are improved and that the conclusions reached from the findings of research studies are valid.

In terms of sex therapy with couples, sufficient studies have now been carried out to enable questions to be answered with some confidence concerning whether one therapist is as effective as two, and what are the most suitable schedule of treatment sessions (Chapter 13). There are, however, several other aspects of sex therapy to which research should be directed, although some findings about them are beginning to emerge. There are many factors in the aetiology of sexual dysfunction which require further examination. The hormonal aspects of sexual problems, especially those of women, are one major area. More efficient and simple means of detecting erectile dysfunction of organic aetiology is another. The pharmacology of sexual arousal and response is a vast but virtually unexplored area. One question which might be examined in this respect is why some people develop sexual side-effects of medication while others do not. Answers to this question might help further our understanding of the causes of sexual disorders of apparently psychogenic origin.

In sex therapy itself there are several important questions which require more attention. The components of treatment should be examined to determine which are most important for which type of client. In other words, how can therapy be best tailored to the particular needs of each person or couple? Self-help treatments could be investigated further, because the great demand for sex therapy necessitates a careful search for brief but effective interventions. Although hormonal and other drug therapies do not seem to have a large role in the treatment of sexual disorders, except when there are obvious deficiency states, their use, possibly in combination with psychological forms of therapy, requires further investigation.

The need for developing effective clinical approaches to the sexual problems associated with physical disability, including those resulting from disorders such as diabetes, has already been emphasized. These approaches also require careful research and evaluation. One sexual dysfunction which often causes great problems for therapists is that of impaired sexual interest, especially in women. Further work is needed to find more effective approaches to this difficult problem.

Although the characteristics of people which are associated with different types of outcome are becoming clearer, there is room for further work in this area. This should allow greater precision in the assessment of people for sex therapy and other forms of help. Finally, much more needs to be known about the long-term outcome of sex therapy, and what approaches provide the best long-term outcome. For example, booster sessions of treatment might be an economical way of preventing relapses in those who are most vulnerable.

CONCLUSIONS

In this final chapter, various important issues in the field of sex therapy have been highlighted. One cannot ignore the importance of cultural attitudes to sexuality, nor the ethical issues in therapy itself, including the necessity to avoid imposition of values and goals. There are sizeable groups of people for whom sex therapy is not at present helpful, and others, such as the disabled, for whom therapy is often unavailable. Services for people with sexual problems are patchy, especially in the UK. Attention needs to be paid to how this situation can be improved. This focuses attention on the need for provision of efficient training resources. The prevention of sexual disorders requires a whole text to itself, because it is so important yet controversial. Adequate and carefully planned sex education and responsible attitudes on the part of the media would represent major improvements in this area. Finally, there are several important and fascinating research needs in this field. If the next few years witness as many important developments in the treatment of sexual problems as have occurred during little more than the past decade, the outlook for people with such problems in future should be even brighter.

Recommended reading

Readers may find the following books useful. They are divided into those which will help extend the reader's knowledge, and those that are useful for recommending to people with sexual problems or people who wish to improve their sexual information. There is also a list of professional journals specializing in papers on sexuality and sexual dysfunction.

Other books which may be of interest to the reader

Arentewicz, G. and Schmidt, G. (eds.) (1983). *The treatment of sexual disorders*. Basic Books, New York. (Includes some interesting research findings concerning sex therapy with couples, and transcripts of therapy sessions.)

Bancroft, J. (1983). *Human sexuality and its problems*. Churchill Livingstone, Edinburgh. (An excellent authoritative account of all the major aspects of human sexuality.)

Elstein, M. (ed.) (1980). *Sexual medicine*. Clinics in Obstetrics and Gynaecology, Vol. 7 (2). Saunders, London.

Greencross, W. (1976). *Entitled to love: the sexual and emotional needs of the handicapped*. Mallaby Press and National Marriage Guidance Council, in association with the National Fund for Research into Crippling Diseases.

Heslinga, K. (1974). *Not made of stone*. Charles Thomas, Illinois. (A clinical approach to the sexual problems of the disabled.)

Kaplan, H. S. (1974). *The new sex therapy*. Baillière Tindall, London. (A detailed account of an eclectic approach to sex therapy.)

Kaplan, H. S. (1976). *The illustrated manual of sex therapy*. Souvenir, London. (A useful summary of this author's approach, and excellent drawings which may be useful in therapy.)

Kolodny, R. C., Masters, W. H., and Johnson, V. E. (1979). *Textbook of sexual medicine*. Little Brown, Boston. (A comprehensive review of the effects on sexual function of physical disorders and their treatments.)

LoPiccolo, J. and LoPiccolo, L. (eds.) (1978). *Handbook of sex therapy.* Plenum, New York. (A useful collection of papers, most of which have been published elsewhere.)

Masters, W. H. and Johnson, V. E. (1966). *Human sexual response.* Little Brown, Boston. (A detailed account based on the authors' original studies of sexual response.)

Masters, W. H. and Johnson, V. E. (1970). *Human sexual inadequacy.* Churchill, London. (The original description of the authors' approach to sex therapy.)

Masters, W. H. and Johnson, V. E. (1979). *Homosexuality in perspective.* Little Brown, Boston. (An account of the sexual response and problems of homosexuals, and sex therapy with homosexual couples.)

Stuart, R. B. (1980). *Helping couples change.* Guilford Press, New York. (A behavioural approach to marital therapy.)

Self-help books which may be recommended to people with sexual problems

Barbach, L. G. (1976). *For yourself: the fulfilment of female sexuality.* Signet, New York. (A self-help guide for women with primary orgasmic dysfunction.)

Felstein, I. (1980). *Sex in later life.* Granada, London. (A general account of sexuality and sexual problems of older people.)

Greenwood, J. (1984). *Coping with sexual relationships.* McDonald, Edinburgh. (Includes advice on solving sexual problems.)

Heiman, J., LoPiccolo, L., and LoPiccolo, J. (1976). *Becoming orgasmic: a sexual growth program for women.* Prentice-Hall, New Jersey. (Another book for women with orgasmic dysfunction.)

Zilbergeld, B. (1980). *Men and sex.* Fontana, London (Includes useful advice for men with sexual problems.)

Sex education books for adults

Delvin, D. (1974). *The book of love.* New English Library, London. (Very useful: deals with many aspects of sexuality and sexual relationships in a pleasantly simple and direct manner.)

Phillips, A. and Rakusen, J. (1978). *Our bodies ourselves.* Penguin, London. (A useful book for women.)

Sex education for young people

Claësson, B. H. (1980). *Boy, girl, man, woman.* Penguin, London.

Kaplan, H. S. (1979). *Making sense of sex.* Quartet, London. (A detailed account of sexuality for the sophisticated teenager.)

Journals specializing in sexuality and sexual dysfunction

Archives of Sexual Behaviour. Plenum, New York.
Journal of Sex and Marital Therapy. Brunner/Mazel, New York.
Journal of Sex Research. Society for the Scientific Study of Sex, New York.
Medical Aspects of Human Sexuality. Hospital Publications, New York.
Sexuality and Disability. Human Sciences Press, New York.
British Journal of Sexual Medicine. Medical News Tribune, London.

(Many other medical, psychiatry and psychology journals also carry occasional papers in this field)

References

Abram, H. S., Hester, L. R., Sheridan, W. F., and Epstein, G. M. (1975). Sexual functioning in patients with chronic renal failure. *Journal of Nervous and Mental Disease*, **160**, 220-6.

Abramov, L. S. (1976). Sexual life and sexual frigidity among women developing acute myocardial infarction. *Psychosomatic Medicine*, **38**, 418-25.

Annon, J. S. (1974). *The behavioural treatment of sexual problems:* Vol. 1: *Brief therapy*. Enabling Systems, Honolulu.

Ansari, J. M. A. (1976). Impotence: prognosis (a controlled study). *British Journal of Psychiatry*, **128**, 194-8.

Arentewicz, G. and Schmidt, G. (eds.) (1983). *The treatment of sexual disorders*. Basic Books, New York.

Azizi, F., Vagenakis, A. G., Longcope, C., Ingbar, S. H., and Braverman, L. E. (1973). Decreased serum testosterone concentration in male heroin and methadone addicts. *Steroids*, **22**, 467-72.

Balint, M. (1955). *The doctor, his patient and the illness*. Pitman Medical, London.

—— and Balint, E. (1961). *Psychotherapeutic techniques in medicine*. Tavistock Publications, London.

Bancroft, J. (1980). Endocrinology of sexual function. In *Sexual medicine* (ed. M. Elstein). Clinics in Obstetrics and Gynaecology, Vol. 7, (2), pp. 253-81. Saunders, London.

—— (1983). *Human sexuality and its problems*. Churchill Livingstone, Edinburgh.

—— and Coles, L. (1976). Three years' experience in a sexual problems clinic. *British Medical Journal*, i, 1575-77.

—— Davidson, D. W., Warner, P., and Tyrer, G. (1980). Androgens and sexual behaviour in women using oral contraceptives. *Clinical Endocrinology*, **12**, 327-40.

Barbach, L. G. (1974). Group treatment of pre-orgasmic women. *Journal of Sex and Marital Therapy*, **1**, 139-45.

—— (1976). *For yourself: the fulfilment of female sexuality.* Signet, New York.

—— (1980). *Women discover orgasm: a therapist's guide to a new treatment approach.* Free Press, New York.

—— and Flaherty, M. (1980). Group treatment of situationally orgasmic women. *Journal of Sex and Marital Therapy,* **6**, 19-29.

Barragry, J. M., Makin, H. L. J., Trafford, D. J. H., and Scott, D. F. (1978). Effects of anticonvulsants on plasma testosterone and sex hormone binding globulin levels. *Journal of Neurology, Neorosurgery and Psychiatry,* **41**, 913-14.

Beaumont, G. (1977). Sexual side effects of clomipramine (Anafranil). *Journal of International Medical Research,* **5**, Suppl. 1, 37-44.

Beaumont, P. J. V., Abraham, S. F., and Simson, K. G. (1981). The psychosexual histories of adolescent girls and young women with anorexia nervosa. *Psychological Medicine,* **11**, 131-40.

—— Beardwood, C. J., and Russell, G. F. M. (1972). The occurrence of the syndrome of anorexia nervosa in male subjects. *Psychological Medicine,* **2**, 216-51.

Beck, A. T. (1967). *Depression: clinical, experimental, and theoretical aspects.* Harper and Row, New York.

—— Rush, A. J., Shaw, B. F., and Emery, G. (1979). *Cognitive Therapy of Depression.* Guilford, New York.

Becker, J. V., Skinner, L. J., Abel, G. G., and Treacey, E. C. (1982). Incidence and types of seasonal dysfunctions in rape and incest victims. *Journal of Sex and Marital Therapy,* **8**, 65-74.

Begg, A., Dickerson, M., and Loudon, N. B. (1976). Frequency of self-reported sexual problems in a family planning clinic. *Journal of Family Planning Doctors,* **2**, 41-8.

Beischer, N. A. (1967). The anatomical and functional results of mediolateral episiotomy. *Medical Journal of Australia,* **2**, 189-95.

Belliveau, F. and Richter, L. (1970). *Understanding human sexual inadequacy.* Coronet, London.

Bergler, E. (1951). *Neurotic counterfeit-sex.* Grune and Stratton, New York.

Blakeney, P., Kinder, B. N., Creson, D., Powell, L. C., and Sutton, C. (1976). A short-term, intensive workshop approach for the treatment of human sexual inadequacy. *Journal of Sex and Marital Therapy,* **2**, 124-9.

Bloch, A., Maeder, J. P., and Haissly, J. C. (1975). Sexual problems after myorcardial infarction. *American Heart Journal,* **90**, 536-7.

Brady, J. P. (1966). Brevital relaxation treatment of frigidity. *Behaviour Research and Therapy,* **4**, 71-8.

British Medical Journal (1979). Drugs and male sexual function. *British Medical Journal,* **2**, 883-4.

Brown, P. and Faulder, C. (1977). *Treat yourself to sex: a guide for good loving*. Dent, London (and (1979): Penguin, London).

Bulpitt, C. J., Dollery, C. T., and Carne, S. (1976). Change in symptoms of hypertensive patients after referral to hospital clinic. *British Heart Journal*, **38**, 121-8.

Burgess, A. W. and Holmstrom, L. L. (1979). Rape: sexual disruption and recovery. *American Journal of Orthopsychiatry*, **49**, 648-57.

Burnap, D. W. and Golden, J. S. (1967). Sexual problems in medical practice. *Journal of Medical Education*, **42**, 673-80.

Burnham, W. R., Lennard-Jones, J. E., and Brooke, B. N. (1976). The incidence and nature of sexual problems among married iliostomists. *Gut*, **17**, 391-2.

Calderone, M. S. (1978). Is sex education preventative? In *The prevention of sexual disorders: issues and approaches* (ed. C. B. Qualls, and J. P. Wincze, and D. H. Barlow). Plenum, New York.

Campbell, I. W., Ewing, D. J., Clarke, B. F., and Duncan, L. J. P. (1974). Testicular pain sensation in diabetic autonomic neuropathy. *British Medical Journal*, **2**, 638-9.

Carney, A., Bancroft, J., and Mathews, A. (1978). Combination of hormonal and psychological treatment for female sexual unresponsiveness: a comparative study. *British Journal of Psychiatry*, **132**, 339-46.

Cartwright, A. (1970). *Parents and family planning services*. Routledge and Kegan Paul, London.

Catalan, J., Bradley, M., Gallwey, J., and Hawton, K. (1981). Sexual dysfunction and psychiatric morbidity in patients attending a clinic for sexually transmitted diseases. *British Journal of Psychiatry*, **138**, 292-6.

Chesney, A. P., Blakeney, P. E., Chan, F. A., and Coley, C. M. (1981). The impact of sex therapy on sexual behaviours and marital communication. *Journal of Sex and Marital Therapy*, **7**, 70-9.

—— —— Cole, C. M., and Chan, F. A. (1981). A comparison of couples who have sought sex therapy with couples who have not. *Journal of Sex and Marital Therapy*, **7**, 131-40.

Christopher, E. (1982). Psychosexual medicine in a mixed racial community. *British Journal of Family Planning*, **7**, 115-19.

Cicero, T. J., Bell, R. D., Wiest, W. G., Allison, J. H., Polakoski, K., and Robins, E. (1975). Function of the male sex organs in heroin and methadone users. *New England Journal of Medicine*, **292**, 882-7.

Clement, U. and Schmidt, G. (1983). The outcome of couple therapy for sexual dysfunctions using three different formats. *Journal of Sex and Marital Therapy*, **9**, 67-78.

Cooper, A. J. (1969). Disorders of sexual potency in the male: a clinical and statistical study of some factors related to short-term prognosis. *British Journal of Psychiatry*, **115**, 709-19.

Cooper, A. J. (1970). Frigidity, treatment and short-term prognosis. *Journal of Psychosomatic Research*, **14**, 133-47.

—— (1974). A blind evaluation of a penile ring—a sex aid for impotent males. *British Journal of Psychiatry*, **124**, 402-6.

—— (1979). A review of 215 cases seen in a sex clinic. *British Journal of Sexual Medicine*, **6** (45), 38-42.

Crisp, A. M. (1967). Anorexia nervosa. *British Journal of Hospital Medicine*, **1**, 713-18.

Crowe, M. J. (1978). Conjoint marital therapy: a controlled outcome study. *Psychological Medicine*, 8, 623-36.

—— Gillan, P., and Golombek, S. (1981). Form and content in the conjoint treatment of sexual dysfunction: a controlled study. *Behaviour Research and Therapy*, **19**, 47-54.

Cushman, P. (1972). Sexual behaviour in heroin addiction and methadone maintenance. *New York State Journal of Medicine*, **72**, 1261-5.

Davidson, J. M., Camargo, C. A., and Smith, E. R. (1979). Effects of androgens on sexual behaviour in hypogonadal men. *Journal of Clinical Endocrinology and Metabolism*, **48**, 955-8.

—— Kwan, M., and Greenleaf, W. J. (1982). Hormonal replacement and sexuality in men. In *Diseases of sex and sexuality* (ed. J. Bancroft). Clinics in Endocrinology and Metabolism, Vol. 11, pp. 599-623. Saunders, London.

Dekker, J. and Everaerd, W. (1983). A long-term follow-up study of couples treated for sexual dysfunctions. *Journal of Sex and Marital Therapy*, **9**, 99-113.

Delvin, D. (1974). *The book of love*. New English Library, London.

Dennerstein, L. and Burrows, G. D. (1982). Hormone replacement therapy and sexuality in women. In *Diseases of sex and sexuality* (ed. J. Bancroft). Clinics in Endocrinology and Metabolism, Vol. 11, pp. 661-79. Saunders, London.

Derogatis, L. R., Meyer, J. K., and King, K. M. (1981). Psychopathology in individuals with sexual dysfunction. *American Journal of Psychiatry*, **138**, 759-63.

Dickinson, R. L. (1933). *Human sex anatomy*. Williams and Wilkins, Baltimore.

—— (1949). *Human sex anatomy*. Williams and Wilkins, Baltimore.

Dow, M. G. T. (1983). A controlled comparative evaluation of conjoint counselling and self-help behavioural treatment for sexual dysfunction. Unpublished Ph.D. Thesis, University of Glasgow.

Duddle, C. M. (1975). The treatment of marital psycho-sexual problems. *British Journal of Psychiatry*, **127**, 169-70.

—— (1977). Etiological factors in the unconsummated marriage. *Journal of Psychosomatic Research,* **21**, 157-60.

—— and Ingram, A. (1980). Treating sexual dysfunction in couples groups. In *Medical sexology* (ed. R. Forleo and W. Pasini), pp. 598-605. Elsevier, North Holland.

Ersner-Hershfield, R. and Kopel, S. (1979). Group treatment of pre-orgasmic women: evaluation of partner involvement and spacing of sessions. *Journal of Consulting and Clinical Psychology,* **47**, 750-9.

Everaerd, W. (1977). Comparative studies of short-term treatment methods for sexual inadequacies. In *Progress in sexology* (ed. R. Gemme and C. C. Wheeler), pp. 153-65. Plenum, New York.

Fairburn, C. G., Wu, F. C. W., McCulloch, D. K., Borsay, D. Q., Ewing, D. J., Clarke, B. F., and Bancroft, J. H. J. (1982). The clinical features of diabetic impotence: a preliminary study. *British Journal of Psychiatry,* **140**, 447-52.

Feldman-Summers, S., Gordon, P. E., and Meagher, J. R. (1979). The impact of rape on sexual satisfaction. *Journal of Abnormal Psychology,* **88**, 101-5.

Finkelhor, D. (1980). Sex among siblings: a survey on prevalence, variety and effects. *Archives of Sexual Behaviour,* **9**, 171-94.

Fisher, S. (1973). *The female orgasm: psychology, physiology, fantasy.* Allen Lane, London.

Fisher, C., Schiavi, R. C., Edwards, A., Davis, D. M., Reitman, M., and Fine, J. (1979). Evaluation of nocturnal penile tumescence in the differential diagnosis of sexual impotence. *Archives of General Psychiatry,* **36**, 431-7.

Fordney-Settlage, D. S. (1975). Heterosexual dysfunction: Evaluation of treatment procedures. *Archives of Sexual Behaviour,* **4**, 367-87.

Forsberg, L., Gustavii, B., Hojerback, T., and Olsson, A. M. (1979). Impotence, smoking and β-blocking drugs. *Fertility and Sterility,* **31**, 589-91.

—— and Olsson, A. M. (1980). Presented at *Second International Conference on Vasculogenic Impotence,* Monaco, 8-12 October. Quoted in Wagner and Green (1981).

Francis, W. H. and Jeffcoate, T. N. A. (1961). Dyspareunia following vaginal operations. *Journal of Obstetrics and Gynaecology of the British Commonwealth,* **68**, 1-10.

Frank, E., Anderson, C., and Kupfer, D. J. (1976). Profiles of couples seeking sex therapy and marital therapy. *American Journal of Psychitry,* **133**, 559-62.

—— —— and Rubinstein, D. (1978). Frequency of sexual dysfunction in "normal" couples. *New England Journal of Medicine,* **299**, 111-15.

Freud, S. (1949). *Three essays on the theory of sexuality.* Imago, London.

Friday, N. (1975). *My secret garden.* Virago, London.

Friedman, D. (1968). The treatment of impotence by brietal relaxation therapy. *Behaviour Research and Therapy,* **6,** 257-61.

Friedman, L. J. (1962). *Virgin wives: a study of unconsummated marriages.* Tavistock Publications, London.

Fritz, G. S., Stoll, K., and Wagner, N. (1981). A comparison of males and females who were sexually molested as children. *Journal of Sex and Marital Therapy,* **7,** 54-9.

Garde, K. and Lunde, I. (1980a). Female sexual behaviour: a study in a random sample of 40-year-old women. *Maturitas,* **2,** 225-40.

—— —— (1980b). Social background and social status: influence on female sexual behaviour. A random sample study of 40-year-old Danish women. *Maturitas,* **2,** 241-6.

Gath, D., Cooper, P., and Day, A. (1982). Hysterectomy and psychiatric disorder: I. Levels of psychiatric morbidity before and after hysterectomy. *British Journal of Psychiatry,* **140,** 335-50.

Gebhard, P. H. and Johnson, A. B. (1979). *The Kinsey data: marginal tabulations of the 1938-1963 interviews conducted by the Institute for Sex Research.* Saunders, Philadelphia.

Goldberg, D. C., Whipple, B., Fishkin, R. E., Waxman, H., Fink, P. J., and Weisberg, M. (1983). The Grafenberg spot and female ejaculation: a review of initial hypotheses. *Journal of Sex and Marital Therapy,* **9,** 27-37.

Golden, J. S., Price, S., Heinrich, A. G., and Lobitz, W. C. (1978). Group vs couple treatment of sexual dysfunctions. *Archives of Sexual Behaviour,* **7,** 593-602.

Gornick, P. (1976). Urologic problems and sexual dysfunction. In *Sex and the life cycle.* (ed. W. W. Oaks, G. A. Melchiode, and I. Ficher) pp. 191-7. Grune and Stratton, New York.

Gossop, M. R., Stern, R., and Connell, P. H. (1974). Drug dependance and sexual function: a comparison of intravenous users of narcotics and oral users of amphetamines. *British Journal of Psychiatry,* **124,** 431-4.

Graber, B. and Kline-Graber, G. (1980). Pathophysiology of pubococcygeus muscle. In *Medical sexology* (ed. R. Forleo and W. Pasini), pp. 267-72. Elsevier, North Holland.

Greenwood, J. (1984). *Coping with sexual relationships.* McDonald, Edinburgh.

Hartman, L. M. (1980). Relationship factors and sexual dysfunction. *Canadian Journal of Psychiatry,* **25,** 560-3.

Haslam, M. T. (1965). The treatment of psychogenic dyspareunia by reciprocal inhibition. *British Journal of Psychiatry,* **111,** 280-2.

Hawton, K. (1980). Training in the management of psychosexual problems. *Medical Education,* **14,** 214-18.

—— (1982). The behavioural treatment of sexual dysfunction. *British*

Journal of Psychiatry, **140**, 94-101.

—— (1983) Prognostic factors in sex therapy. Unpublished paper presented to the Ninth Annual Meeting of the International Academy of Sex Research, New York.

—— (1984). Sexual adjustment of men who have had strokes. *Journal of Psychosomatic Research*, **28**, 243-9.

Heiman, J. R. and LoPiccolo, J. (1983). Clinical outcome of sex therapy. *Archives of General Psychiatry*, **40**, 443-9.

—— LoPiccolo, L., and LoPiccolo, J. (1976). *Becoming orgasmic: a sexual growth program for women*. Prentice-Hall, New Jersey.

Heisler, J. (1983). *Sexual therapy in the National Marriage Guidance Council*. Marriage Guidance Council, Rugby.

Herzberg, B. N., Draper, K. C., Johnson, A. L., and Nicol, G. C. (1971). Oral contraceptives, depression and libido. *British Medical Journal*, **3**, 495-500.

Heslinga, K. (1974). *Not made of stone*. Charles Thomas, Illinois.

Higgins, G. E. (1978). Aspects of sexual response in adults with spinal-cord injury: a review of the literature. In *Handbook of sex therapy* (ed. J. LoPiccolo and L. LoPiccolo), pp. 387-410. Plenum, New York.

Hite, S. (1976). *The Hite report: a nationwide study of female sexuality*. Dell, New York.

Jensen, S. B. (1979). Sexual customs and dysfunction in alcoholics: Part I and Part II. *British Journal of Sexual Medicine*, **6** (53), 29-32; **6** (54), 30-4.

—— (1981). Diabetic sexual dysfunction: a comparative study of 160 insulin treated diabetic men and women and an age-matched control. *Archives of Sexual Behaviour*, **10**, 493-504.

Kalliomaki, J. L., Markkanen, T. K., and Mustonen, V. A. (1961). Sexual behaviour after cerebral vascular accidents. *Fertility and Sterility*, **12**, 156-8.

Kaplan, H. S. (1974). *The new sex therapy*. Baillière Tindall, London.

—— (1976). *The illustrated manual of sex therapy*. Souvenir Press, London.

—— (1977). Hypoactive sexual desire. *Journal of Sex and Marital Therapy*, **3**, 3-9.

—— (1979). *Disorder of sexual desire and other new concepts and techniques in sex therapy*. Brunner/Mazel, New York.

—— Kohl, R. N., Pomeroy, W. B., and Offit, A. K. (1974). Group treatment of premature ejaculation. *Archives of Sexual Behaviour*, **3**, 443-52.

Kegel, A. H. (1952). Sexual function of the pubococcygeus muscle. *Western Journal of Surgery, Obstetrics and Gynaecology*, **60**, 521-4.

Kinsey, A. C., Pomeroy, W. B., and Martin, C. E. (1948). *Sexual behaviour in the human male*. Saunders, Philadelphia.

—— —— and Gebhard, P. H. (1953). *Sexual behaviour in the human female*. Saunders, Philadelphia.

Kockott, G., Dittmar, F., and Nusselt, L. (1975). Systematic desensitization of erectile impotence: a controlled study. *Archives of Sexual Behaviour*, **4**, 493-500.

Kolodny, R. C. (1971). Sexual dysfunction in diabetic females. *Diabetes*, **20**, 557-9.

—— Masters, W. H., Kolodner, R. M., and Toro, G. (1974). Depression of plasma testosterone levels after chronic intensive marihuana use. *New England Journal of Medicine*, **290**, 872-4.

—— —— and Johnson, V. E. (1979). *Textbook of sexual medicine*, Little Brown, Boston.

Krop, H., Hall, D., and Mehta, J. (1979). Sexual concerns after myocardial infarction. *Sexuality and Disability*, **2**, 91-7.

Ladas, A. K., Whipple, B., and Perry, J. D. (1982). *The G spot and other recent discoveries about human sexuality*. Holt, Rinehart and Winston, New York.

The Lancet (1981). Adverse reactions to bendrofluazide and propranolol for the treatment of mild hypertension. *Lancet*, **ii**, 539-43.

Lansky, M .R. and Davenport, A. E. (1975). Difficulties in brief conjoint treatment of sexual dysfunction. *American Journal of Psychiatry*, **132**, 177-9.

Lazarus, A. A. (1963). The treatment of chronic frigidity by systematic desensitization. *Journal of Nervous and Mental Disease*, **136**, 272-8.

Leiblum, S. R. and Ersner-Hershfield, R. (1977). Sexual enhancement groups for dysfunctional women: an evaluation. *Journal of sex and Marital Therapy*, **3**, 139-52.

—— and Rosen, R. C. (1979). The weekend workshop for dysfunctional couples: assets and limitations. *Journal of Sex and Marital Therapy*, **5**, 57-69.

—— —— and Pierce, D. (1976). Group treatment format: mixed sexual dysfunctions. *Archives of Sexual Behaviour*, **5**, 313-22.

Lemere, F. and Smith, J. W. (1973). Alcohol-induced sexual impotence. *American Journal of Psychiatry*, **130**, 212-13.

Levay, A. N. and Kagle, A. (1977). A study of treatment needs following sex therapy. *American Journal of Psychiatry*, **134**, 970-3.

Levin, R. J. (1980). Physiology of sexual function in women. In *Sexual medicine* (ed. M. Elstein). Clinics in Obstetrics and Gynaecology, Vol. 7, pp. 213-52. Saunders, London.

Levine, S. B. and Agle, D. (1978). The effectiveness of sex therapy for chronic secondary impotence. *Journal of Sex and Marital Therapy*, **4**, 235-8.

—— and Yost, M. A. (1976). Frequency of sexual dysfunction in a general gynaecological clinic: an epidemiological approach. *Archives of Sexual Behaviour*, **5**, 229-38

Lilius, H. G., Valtonen, E. J., and Wikström, J. (1976). Sexual problems in patients suffering from multiple sclerosis. *Journal of Chronic Diseases*, **29**, 643-7.

Lobitz, W. C. and Baker, E. L. (1979). Group treatment of single males with erectile dysfunction. *Archives of Sexual Behaviour*, **8**, 127-38.

LoPiccolo, J. (1983). Co-therapy versus single therapy (personal communication).

—— and Lobitz, W. C. (1972). The role of masturbation in the treatment of orgasmic dysfunction. *Archives of Sexual Behaviour*, **2**, 163-71.

—— and Steger, J. C. (1974). The sexual interaction inventory: a new instrument for the assessment of sexual dysfunction. *Archives of Sexual Behaviour*, **3**, 585-95.

Lowe, J. C. and Mikulas, W. L. (1975). Use of written material in learning self-control of premature ejaculation. *Psychological Reports*, **37**, 295-8.

Lundberg, P. O. (1980). Sexual dysfunction in women with multiple sclerosis. In *Medical sexology*. (ed. R. Forleo and W. Pasini), pp. 426-9. Elsevier, North Holland.

Lyketsos, G. C., Sakka, P., and Mailis, A. (1983). The sexual adjustment of chronic schizophrenics: a preliminary study. *British Journal of Psychiatry*, **143**, 376-82.

McCulloch, D. K., Campbell, I. W., Wu, F. C., Prescott, R. J. and Clarke, B. F. (1980). The prevalence of diabetic impotence. *Diabetologia*, **18**, 279-83.

McGovern, K. P., Kirkpatrick, C. C., and LoPiccolo, J. (1976). A behavioural group treatment program for sexually dysfunctional couples. *Journal of Marital and Family Counseling*, **2**, 397-404.

—— Stewart, R. C., and LoPiccolo, J. (1975). Secondary orgasmic dysfunction. I: Analysis and strategies for treatment, *Archives of Sexual Behaviour*, **4**, 265-75.

McMullen, S. and Rosen, R. C. (1979). Self-administered masturbation training in the treatment of primary orgasmic dysfunction. *Journal of Consulting and Clinical Psychology*, **47**, 912-18.

McNab, D. and Hawton, K. (1981). Disturbances of sex hormones in anorexia nervosa in the male. *Postgraduate Medical Journal*, **57**, 254-6.

Maguire, G. P., Lee, E. G., Bevington, D. J., Küchemann, C. S.

Crabtree, R. J., and Cornell, C. E. (1978). Psychiatric problems in the first year after mastectomy. *British Medical Journal,* **1**, 963-5.

Masters, W. H. and Johnson, V. E. (1966). *Human sexual response.* Churchill, London.

—— and —— (1970). *Human sexual inadequacy.* Churchill, London.

—— and —— (1979). *Homosexuality in perspective.* Little Brown, Boston.

Mathew, R. J. and Weinman, M. L. (1982). Sexual dysfunctions in depression. *Archives of Sexual Behaviour,* **11**, 323-8.

Mathews, A., Bancroft, J., Whitehead, A., Hackmann, A., Julier, D., Bancroft, J., Gath, D., and Shaw, P. (1976). The behavioural treatment of sexual inadequacy: a comparative study. *Behaviour Research and Therapy,* **14**, 427-36.

—— Whitehead, A., and Kellett, J. (1983). Psychological and hormonal factors in the treatment of female sexual dysfunction. *Psychological Medicine,* **13**, 83-92.

Maurice, W. L. and Guze, S. B. (1970). Sexual dysfunction and associated psychiatric disorders. *Comprehensive Psychiatry,* **11**, 539-43.

Mehta, J. and Krop, H. (1979). The effect of myocardial infarction on sexual functioning. *Sexuality and Disability,* **2**, 115-21.

Mendelson, J. H., Kuehnle, J., Ellingboe, J., and Babor, T. F. (1974). Plasma testosterone levels before, during and after chronic marihuana smoking. *New England Journal of Medicine,* **291**, 1051-5.

Meyer, J. K., Schmidt, C. W., Lucas, M. J., and Smith, E. (1975). Short-term treatment of sexual problems: interim report. *American Journal of Psychiatry,* **132**, 172-6

Michal, V. (1982). Arterial disease as a cause of impotence. In *Diseases of sex and sexuality* (ed. J. Bancroft). Clinics in Endocrinology and Metabolism, Vol. 11, pp. 725-48. Saunders, London.

Mills, K. H. and Kilmann, P. R. (1982). Group treatment of sexual dysfunctions: a methodological review of the outcome literature. *Journal of Sex and Marital Therapy,* **8**, 259-96.

Milne, H. B. (1976). The role of the psychiatrist. In *Psychosexual Problems* (ed. H. Milne, and S. J. Hardy), pp. 65-87. Bradford University Press.

Mrazek, P. B. and Mrazek, D. A. (1981). The effects of child sexual abuse; methodological considerations. In *Sexually abused children and their families* (ed. P. B. Mrazek and C. H. Kempe), pp. 235-45. Pergamon, Oxford.

Munjack, D., Cristol, A., Goldstein, A., Phillips, D., Goldberg, A., Whipple, K., Staples, F., and Kanno, P. (1976). Behavioural treatment of orgasmic dysfunction: a controlled study. *British Journal of Psychiatry,* **129**, 497-502.

Nairne, K. D. and Hemsley, D. R. (1983). The use of directed masturbation training in the treatment of primary anorgasmia. *British Journal of Clinical Psychology*, **22**, 283-94.

Nettelbladt, P. and Uddenberg, N. (1979). Sexual dysfunction and sexual satisfaction in 58 married Swedish men. *Journal of Psychosomatic Research*, **23**, 141-7.

O'Connor, J. F. (1976). Sexual problems, therapy, and prognostic factors. In *Clinical management of sexual disorders* (ed. J. K. Meyer), pp. 74-98. Williams and Wilkins, Baltimore.

—— and Stern, L. O. (1972). Developmental factors in functional sexual disorders. *New York State Journal of Medicine*, **72**, 1838-43.

Perlman, S. D. and Abramson, P. R. (1982). Sexual satisfaction among married and cohabiting individuals. *Journal of Consulting and Clinical Psychology*, **50**, 458-460.

Persson, G. (1980). Sexuality in a 70-year-old urban population. *Journal of Psychosomatic Research*, **24**, 335-42.

Phillips, A. and Rakusen, J. (1971). *Our bodies ourselves.* Boston Women's Health Collective, Boston (also published by Penguin, London (1978)).

Pirke, K. M. and Kockott, G. (1982). Endocrinology of sexual dysfunction. In *Diseases of sex and sexuality* (ed. J. Bancroft). Clinics in Endocrinology and Metabolism, Vol. 11, pp. 625-37. Saunders, London.

Price, S. C., Reynolds, B. S., Cohen, B. D., Anderson, A. J., and Schochet, B. V. (1981). Group treatment of erectile dysfunction for men without partners: a controlled evaluation. *Archives of Sexual Behaviour*, **10**, 253-68.

Renshaw, D. C. (1978). Impotence in diabetics. In *Handbook of sex therapy* (ed. J. LoPiccolo and L. LoPiccolo), pp. 433-40. Plenum, New York.

Rhodes, P. (1975). Sex aids. *British Medical Journal*, **3**, 93-5.

Riley, A. J. and Riley, E. J. (1978). A controlled study to evaluate directed masturbation in the management of primary orgasmic failure in women. *British Journal of Psychiatry*, **133**, 404-9.

Rimm, D. C. and Masters, J. C. (1979). *Behaviour therapy: techniques and empirical findings.* Academic Press, New York.

Roughan, P. A. and Kunst, L. (1981). Do pelvic floor exercises really improve orgasmic potential? *Journal of Sex and Marital Therapy*, **7**, 223-9.

Royal College of General Practitioners (1974). *Oral contraceptives and health.* Pitman, London.

Rubin, A. and Babbot, D. (1958). Impotence and diabetes mellitus. *Journal of the American Medical Association*, **168**, 498-500.

Salmon, U. J. and Geist, S. H. (1943). The effects of androgens upon libido in women. *Journal of Clinical Endocrinology*, **3**, 235-8.

Sanders, D. and Bancroft, J. (1982). Hormones and the sexuality of women—the menstrual cycle. In *Diseases of sex and fertility* (ed. J. Bancroft). Clinics in Endocrinology and Metabolism, Vol. 11, pp. 639-59. Saunders, London.

Schiavi, R. C. (1980). Psychological treatment of erectile distorders in diabetic patients. *Annals of Internal Medicine,* **92,** 337-9.

Scott, D. F. (1978). Sexual functioning in epilepsy. *British Journal of Sexual Medicine,* **5,** 17-18.

Segraves, R. T. (1977). Pharmacological agents causing sexual dysfunction. *Journal of Sex and Marital Therapy,* **3,** 157-76.

Semans, J. M. (1956). Premature ejaculation: a new approach. *Southern Medical Journal,* **49,** 353-7.

Silver, J. R. and Owens, E. (1975). Sexual problems in disorders of the nervous system: II. Psychological reactions. *British Medical Journal,* **3,** 532-4.

Siroky, M. B., Sax, D. S., and Krane, R. J. (1979). Sacral signal tracing: the electrophysiology of the bulbocavernosus reflex. *Journal of Urology,* **122,** 661-4.

Skakkebaek, N. E., Bancroft, J., Davidson, D. W., and Warner, P. M. (1981). Androgen replacement with oral testosterone undeconoate in hypogonadal men: a double-blind controlled study. *Clinical Endocrinology,* **14,** 49-61.

Snyder, D. C. and Berg, P. (1983). Predicting couples' response to brief directive sex therapy. *Journal of Sex and Marital Therapy,* **9,** 114-20.

Spark, R. F., White, R. A., and Connolly, P. B. (1980). Impotence is not always psychogenic. *Journal of the American Medical Association,* **243,** 750-5.

Steele, T. E., Finkelstein, S. H., and Finkelstein, F. O. (1976). Haemodialysis patients and spouses: marital discord, sexual problems, and depression. *Journal of Nervous and Mental Disease,* **162,** 225-37.

Stewart, W. F. R. (1978). Sexual fulfilment for the handicapped. *British Journal of Hospital Medicine,* **20,** 676-80.

Stoll, K. A. B. (1978). Factors affecting outcome in the treatment of sexual dysfunction. Unpublished M.Phil. thesis, London University.

Story, N. L. (1974). Sexual dysfunction resulting from drug side effects. *Journal of Sex Research,* **10,** 132-49.

Stuart, R. B. (1980). *Helping couples change.* Guildford, New York.

Swan, M. and Wilson, L. J. (1979). Sexual and marital problems in a psychiatric out-patient population. *British Journal of Psychiatry,* **135,** 310-14.

Tavris, C. and Sadd, S. (1977). *The redbook report on female sexuality.* Delacorte Press, New York.

Taylor, D. C. (1969). Sexual behaviour and temporal lobe epilepsy. *Archives of Neurology,* **21,** 510-16.

Thorner, M. O. and Besser, G. M. (1977). Hyperprolactinaemia and gonadal function. In *Prolactin and human reproduction* (ed. P. G. Crosignami and C. Robyn), pp. 285-301. Academic Pres, London.

Thornes, B. and Collard, J. (1979). *Who divorces?* Routledge and Kegan Paul, London.

Toone, B., Wheeler, M., and Fenwick, P.(1982). Effects of anticonvulsant drugs on male sex hormones and sexual arousal. In *Psychopharmacology of anticonvulsants* (ed. M. Sandler), pp. 136-42. Oxford University Press.

Tsai, M., Feldman-Summers, S., and Edgar, M. (1979). Childhood molestation: variables related to differential impacts on psychosexual functioning in adult women. *Journal of Abnormal Psychology,* **88,** 407-17.

Tuttle, W., Cook, W., and Fitch, E. (1964). Sexual behaviour in postmyocardial infarction patients. *American Journal of Cardiology,* **13,** 140.

Uddenberg, N. (1974). Psychological aspects of sexual inadequacy in women. *Journal of Psychosomatic Research,* **18,** 33-47.

Van de Velde, T. H. (1930). *Ideal marriage.* Random House, New York.

Van Thiel, D. H. and Lester, R. (1976). Sex and alcohol: a second peak. *New England and Journal of Medicine,* **295,** 835-6.

—— and —— (1979). The effect of chronic alcohol abuse on sexual function. *Clinics in Endocrinology and Metabolism,* **8,** 499-510.

Vas, C. J. (1978). Sexual impotence and some autonomic disturbances in men with multiple sclerosis. In *Sexual consequences of disability* (ed. A. Comfort), pp. 45-60. Stickley, Philadelphia.

Victor, A., Lundberg, P. O., and Johansson, E. D. B. (1977). Induction of sex hormone binding globulin by phenytoin. *British Medical Journal,* **2,** 934-5.

Vinarova, E., Uhlir, O., Skitka, L., and Vinar, O. (1972). Side effects of lithium administration. *Activitas Nervosa Superior,* **14,** 105-7.

Wabrek, A. J. and Burchell, R. C. (1980). Male sexual dysfunction asociated with coronary heart disease. *Archives of Sexual Behaviour,* **9,** 69-75.

Wagner, G. (1981a). Erection: physiology and endocrinology. In *Impotence: physiological, psychological, surgical diagnosis and treatment* (ed. G. Wagner and R. Green), pp. 25-36. Plenum, New York.

—— (1981b). Methods for differential diagnosis of psychogenic and organic erectile failure. In *Impotence: physiological, psychological, surgical diagnosis and treatment* (ed. G. Wagner and R. Green), pp. 89-130. Plenum, New York.

—— (1981c). Surgical treatment of erectile failure. In *Impotence: physiological, psychological, surgical diagnosis and treatment* (ed. G. Wagner and R. Green), pp. 155-66. Plenum, New York.

—— and Green, R. (1981). *Impotence: physiological, psychological, surgical diagnosis and treatment.* Plenum, New York.

—— and Metz, P. (1981). Arteriosclerosis and erectile failure. In *Impotence: physiological, surgical diagnosis, and treatment* (ed. G. Wagner and R. Green), pp. 63-72. Plenum, New York.

Wallace, D. M. and Barbach, L. G. (1974). Preorgasmic group treatment. *Journal of Sex and Marital Therapy*, **1**, 146-54.

Watson, J. P. and Brockman, B. (1982). A follow-up of couples attending a psychosexual problems clinic. *British Journal of Clinical Psychology*, **21**, 143-4.

Weissman, M. M. and Paykel, E. S. (1974). *The depressed woman: a study of social relationships.* University of Chicago Press.

Whitehead, A. and Mathews, A. (1977). Attitude change during behavioural treatment of sexual inadequacy. *British Journal of Social and Clinical Psychology*, **16**, 275-81.

Whitehead, A. and Mathews, A. (1981). Factors in the treatment of sexually unresponsive women. Unpublished paper presented to the Annual Meeting of the British Association for Behavioural Psychotherapy, Bristol.

Wincze, J. P. and Caird, W. K. (1976). The effects of systematic desensitization and video desensitization in the treatment of essential sexual dysfunction in women. *Behaviour Therapy*, **7**, 335-42.

Winokur, G., Clayton, P. J., and Reich, T. (1969). *Manic depressive illness.* Mosby, St. Louis.

Wolpe, J. (1958). *Psychotherapy by reciprocal inhibition.* Stanford University Press, Stanford.

Wright, J., Perreault, R., and Mathieu, M. (1977). The treatment of sexual dysfunction. *Archives of General Psychiatry*, **34**, 881-90.

Zeiss, R. A. (1978). Self-directed treatment for premature ejaculation. *Journal of Consulting and Clinical Psychology*, **46**, 1234-41.

—— Christensen, A., and Levine, A. G. (1978). Treatment for premture ejaculation through male-only groups. *Journal of Sex and Marital Therapy*, **4**, 139-43.

Zilbergeld, B. (1975). Group treatment of sexual dysfunction in men without partners. *Journal of Sex and Marital Therapy*, **1**, 204-14.

—— (1978). *Men and sex.* Little Brown, Boston (and (1980): Fontana, London).

—— and Evans, M. (1980). The inadequacy of Masters and Johnson. *Psychology Today*, August, 29-43.

Index